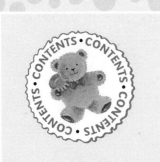

Speech and language difficulties

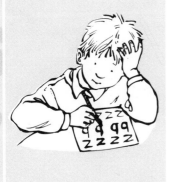

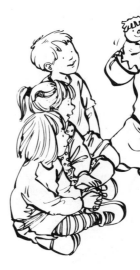

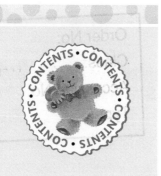
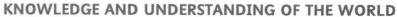

KNOWLEDGE AND UNDERSTANDING OF THE WORLD

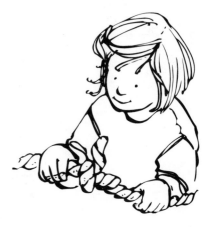

PHYSICAL DEVELOPMENT

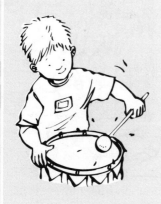

CREATIVE DEVELOPMENT

PHOTOCOPIABLES

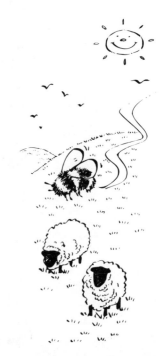

£15·00

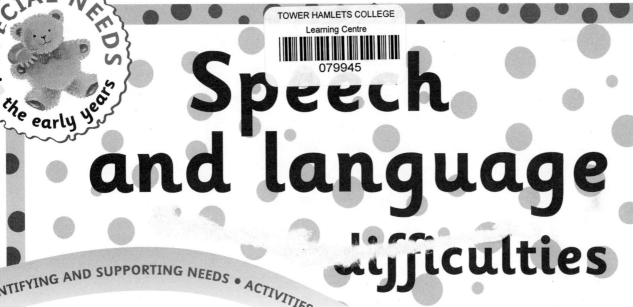

Speech and language *difficulties*

SPECIAL NEEDS in the early years

IDENTIFYING AND SUPPORTING NEEDS • ACTIVITIES COVERING EARLY LEARNING GOALS • WORKING WITH PARENTS

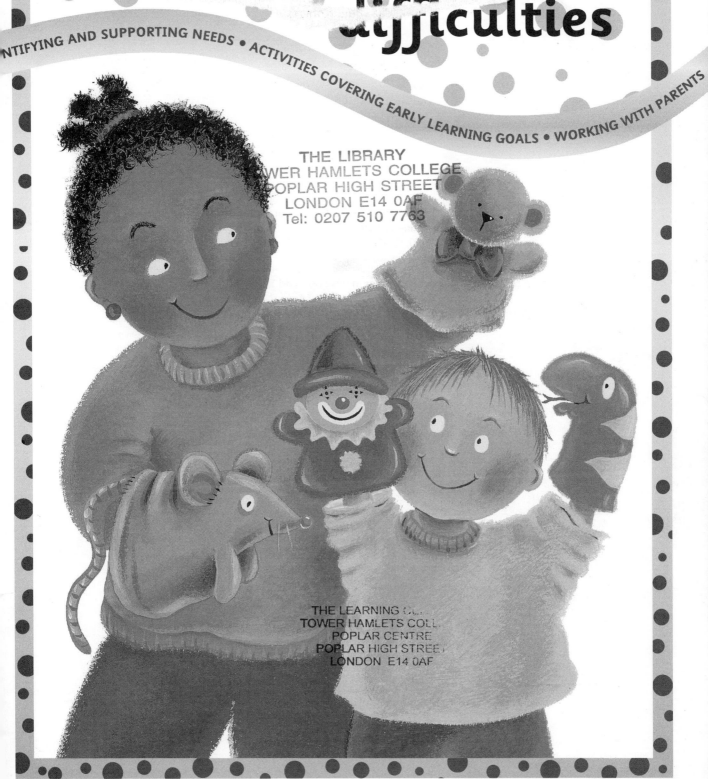

DR HANNAH MORTIMER

Author
Dr Hannah Mortimer

Editor
Lesley Sudlow

Assistant Editor
Saveria Mezzana

Series Designers
Sarah Rock/Anna Oliwa

Designer
Paul Roberts

Illustrations
Shelagh McNicholas

Cover artwork
Claire Henley

Acknowledgements
The publishers gratefully acknowledge permission to reproduce the following
copyright material:

Qualifications and Curriculum Authority for the use of extracts from the
QCA/DfEE document *Curriculum Guidance for the Foundation Stage*
© 2000, Qualifications and Curriculum Authority.

The publishers wish to thank Makaton Vocabulary Development Project for their help in
reproducing the Makaton illustrations in this book, and Sinnington Playgroup for their idea
on page 34.
Every effort has been made to trace copyright holders and the publishers apologize for any
inadvertent omissions.

Text © 2002, Hannah Mortimer
© 2002, Scholastic Ltd

Designed using Adobe Pagemaker

Published by Scholastic Ltd, Villiers House,
Clarendon Avenue, Leamington Spa, Warwickshire CV32 5PR

Visit our website at www.scholastic.co.uk

Printed by Alden Group Ltd, Oxford

3 4 5 6 7 8 9 0   3 4 5 6 7 8 9 0 1

British Library Cataloguing-in-Publication Data A catalogue record for this book is
available from the British Library.

ISBN 0 439 01832 3

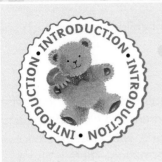

INTRODUCTION

Language and thought are both important features of early learning. When children's speech and language do not develop normally, it is necessary to identify and support their difficulties as soon as possible.

The aims of the series

There is now a new, revised *Code of Practice* for the identification and assessment of special educational needs. This series aims to provide guidance to early years practitioners on how to meet and monitor special educational needs (SEN) under the new Code. The QCA document *Curriculum Guidance for the Foundation Stage* emphasizes the key role that early years practitioners play in identifying needs and responding quickly to them. While most of us feel that an inclusive approach is the best one for all the children concerned, we still need guidance on what an inclusive early years curriculum might actually 'look like' in practice.

Within this series, there are books to help children with most kinds of special needs:

- speech and language difficulties
- behavioural and emotional difficulties
- learning difficulties
- physical and co-ordination difficulties
- medical difficulties
- autistic spectrum difficulties
- sensory difficulties.

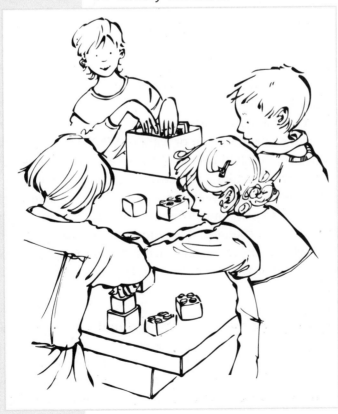

There is also a handbook for the whole series called *Special Needs Handbook*. This provides general guidance and more detail on how to assess, plan for, teach and monitor children with SEN in early years settings.

Many early years groups will, at some point, include children who have speech and language difficulties. Even if children have other kinds of learning difficulties, there is often a difficulty or delay in acquiring language as well. This book will help all early years professionals to recognize and understand such difficulties and to provide inclusive activities for those children concerned. Market research has shown that early years practitioners would

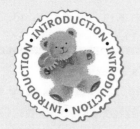

welcome practical advice and guidelines for children with speech and language difficulties.

How to use this book

Chapter 1 gives an introduction to the requirements under the revised *Code of Practice* for SEN as it relates to children who have speech and language difficulties. This is only a brief guide, with close reference made to the series handbook for more information. There is also a reminder of the requirements of the QCA Early Learning Goals and Curriculum Guidelines, with particular reference to those in the area of Communication, language and literacy.

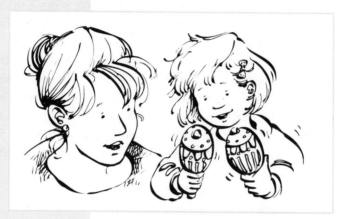

The need for individual education plans for those children who have SEN is introduced and advice is given on how to meet SEN in an inclusive way. There are pointers for developing positive partnership and relationships with parents and carers. Some of the outside agencies that you may be required to liaise with are also mentioned.

Chapter 2 looks more closely at the needs of children who have speech and language difficulties. It gives advice on looking for special opportunities for promoting speech and language development, linked to the Early Years curriculum. Encouragement is given to try a range of approaches and make the use of the full range of resources and activities available in your setting.

Chapters 3 to 8 are activity chapters, each related to one of the QCA Areas of Learning: Personal, social and emotional development; Communication, language and literacy; Mathematical development; Knowledge and understanding of the world; Physical development and Creative development.

Every chapter contains ten activities, each with a learning objective for all the children (with or without SEN) and an individual learning target for any child who might have any one of a range of speech and language difficulties. The activities target different kinds of difficulties in the hope that early years workers will become able to develop a flexible approach to planning inclusive activities, dipping into the ideas which pepper these chapters. It is suggested that you read through them all for their general ideas, and then dip into the activities as and when you need them as part of your general curriculum planning.

Dip-in ideas

Each activity includes a suggestion for the appropriate size of group, a list of what you need, a description of what to do, any special support that might be necessary for a child with special needs, ideas for extending the activity for more able children and suggestions for links with home. Again, these guidelines are flexible and you should take into account the needs of the children in your particular setting.

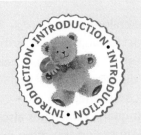

Though this book relates to the early years and SEN procedures followed in England, the general guidance on individual planning, positive behaviour management and activities will be equally relevant to early years workers in other countries.

How children's speech and language normally develop

Children appear to acquire language and speech in a remarkably uniform way and seem to be almost 'pre-programmed' to acquire speech sounds, grammar, meaning and to want to communicate socially. Typically, there is a gradual progression from the first repeated babbling sounds ('bu-bu-bu', 'ma-ma-ma') to single words used with real intent ('mama!', 'dada!'). In time, children build up to two- or three-word phrases. Action words and pronouns begin to develop ('dada gone!', 'me do it!').

Gradually, over the first five years, these phrases build into whole sentences complete with labelling words, action words and describing words. Negatives begin to appear ('not bedtime') and questions begin to be asked, usually with amazing persistence and repetition. The whole of the child's language appears geared towards helping them to find out as much as possible about the world. As they find out more, and develop their language skills, they become able to 'internalize' their language so that thinking, reasoning and predicting inside their head becomes possible.

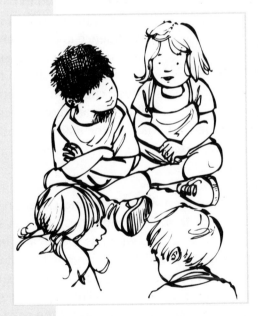

Children with speech and language difficulties

For some children, the above does not happen spontaneously. Perhaps the child is slow to develop all the speech sounds necessary to make clear speech. Most children have immaturities in the way that they speak, for example, 'aminal' instead of 'animal', but these sort themselves out with practice and experience. Some children lack the ability to make certain sounds or cannot co-ordinate the sounds in the required sequence. These children are sometimes described as having 'dyspraxic', 'dysarthric' or 'articulation' difficulties.

For other children, language remains rather like a telegram because they do not naturally acquire the grammar and 'order' that language usually follows. Sometimes this is because their language development is delayed but nevertheless progressing along normal lines. Perhaps these children are delayed in other areas of their development as well and the language delay is just one part of this immaturity.

Some children have a 'specific language disorder' or 'difficulty' which means that they would benefit from specialist therapy and approaches. It is called a 'specific' difficulty because, although the child's language is disordered or delayed, their general intelligence and ability might be

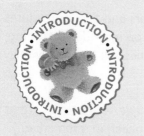
average or even high for their age. For these children, their understanding of language, especially abstract language such as 'big', 'empty' and other concept words, is usually affected as well as their use of language. You might hear these children described as having difficulties in language 'expression' and/or 'comprehension'.

Quite often, children who have specific language difficulties also have difficulties in understanding social situations, in seeing the other point of view, in using their imaginations and in handling conversations. Sometimes these children are described as having 'pragmatic' difficulties. Children with 'semantic and pragmatic' language difficulties have difficulties both in the understanding of abstract language and in the social use of language. *Autistic Spectrum Difficulties* is another book in this series which gives more ideas on helping children with pragmatic difficulties.

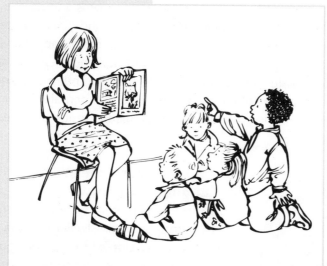

Using resources

The activities described in this book encourage you to make use of a wide range of resources and materials available in your setting. There are ideas for art and craft, story time, physical play, exploring and finding out. Special use is made of circle-time approaches with young children since these have been shown to be very effective in building the children's self-esteem and confidence and in teaching them how to join in and volunteer language within a group.

Research has shown that using a regular music circle time can enhance looking, listening and confidence both within the circle time and beyond. Many of the activities presented in this book use a musical approach.

Links with home

All the activities suggest ways of keeping closely in touch with home. By sharing activities with parents and carers, you can also play a role in helping the carers of a child who has speech and language difficulties to follow approaches that will make everyone feel a lot more encouraged at home. If, in turn, you can encourage carers to share their own expertise and knowledge of their children with you, then you can make your teaching more carefully targeted for the child.

Providing special support

Make sure that the child with SEN is accessing the full range of your early years provision. Clearly this cannot happen if the child is isolated in any way or withdrawn from the group regularly, and this is another reason for collecting ideas for 'inclusive' group activities. 'Support' does not mean individual one-to-one attention. Instead, it can mean playing alongside a child or watching so as to encourage new language and understanding, staying one step ahead of any learning opportunities and teaching the child social skills in small groups.

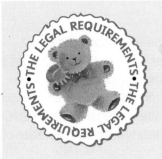

THE LEGAL REQUIREMENTS

This chapter explains the SEN *Code of Practice*, the requirements of the Early Learning Goals and why there is a need for individual education plans for SEN children. There is also practical advice on working with parents and working with outside agencies.

The Code of Practice

The SEN *Code of Practice* is a guide for school governors, registered early years providers and local education authorities, relating to the practical help that they can give to children with special educational needs. It recommends that schools and early years providers should identify the children's needs and take action to meet those needs as early as possible, working together with the carers. The aim is to enable all children with SEN to reach their full potential, to be included fully in their school communities and to make a successful transition to adulthood. The Code gives guidance to schools and early years providers, but it does not tell them what they must do in every case.

The contents of the new, revised SEN *Code of Practice* are described in more detail in the series handbook *Special Needs Handbook*.

The underlying principles for early years settings

All young children have a right to a broad and balanced curriculum which enables them to make maximum progress towards the Early Learning Goals. Early years practitioners must recognize, identify and meet SEN within their settings. There will be a range of provision to meet that need. Most children with SEN will be in a local mainstream early years group or class, even those who have 'statements of SEN'. Parents, children, early years settings and support services should work as partners in planning for and meeting SEN.

The *Code of Practice* is designed to enable SEN to be identified early and addressed. These SEN will normally be met in the local mainstream setting, though some children may need extra consideration or help to be able to access the early years curriculum fully. There is more detailed information about your requirements under the SEN *Code of Practice* in the series handbook. It is recognized that good practice can take many forms and early years providers are encouraged to adopt a flexible and graduated response to the SEN of individual children. This approach recognizes that there is a continuum of SEN and, where necessary, brings increasing specialist expertise on board if the child is experiencing continuing difficulties.

Once a child's SEN have been identified, the providers should intervene through Early Years Action. Each setting should appoint a Special Educational Needs Co-ordinator (SENCO), whose role will be to co-ordinate the special needs provision and act as a point of contact and training for special educational needs.

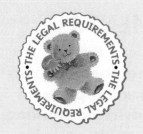

Early Years Action Plus

When reviewing the child's progress and the help that they are receiving, the provider might decide to seek alternative approaches to learning, through the support of the outside support services. These interventions are known as 'Early Years Action Plus'. This is characterized by the involvement of specialists from outside the setting. The SENCO continues to take a leading role, working closely with the member of staff responsible for the child as well as:

● drawing on the advice from outside specialists, for example, speech and language therapists, early years support teachers or educational psychologists

● making sure that the child and his or her carers are consulted and kept informed

● ensuring that an individual education plan (IEP) is drawn up, incorporating the specialist advice, and that it is incorporated within the curriculum planning for the whole setting

● monitoring and reviewing the child's progress with outside specialists

● keeping the head of the setting informed.

For very few children, the help provided by Early Years Action Plus will still not be sufficient to ensure satisfactory progress, even when it has run over several review periods. The provider, external professional and parents may then decide to ask the LEA to consider carrying out a statutory assessment of the child's SEN. The LEA must decide quickly whether or not it has the 'evidence' to indicate that a statutory

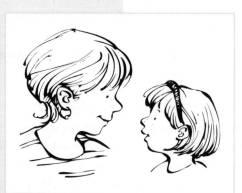

assessment is necessary for a child. It is then responsible for co-ordinating a statutory assessment and will call for the various reports that it requires from the early years teacher (usually a support teacher, early years practitioner or LEA nursery teacher); an educational psychologist; a doctor (who will also gather 'evidence' from any speech and language therapist involved) and the social services department (if involved). It will also ask parents to submit their own views and evidence.

Once the LEA has collected in the evidence, it might decide to issue a 'statement of SEN' for the child. Only children with severe and long-standing SEN will go on to receive a statement – about two per cent of all children. There are various rights of appeal in the cases of disagreement, and the LEA can provide information about these.

Requirements of the Early Learning Goals

Registered early years providers are expected to deliver a broad and balanced curriculum across the six Areas of Learning as defined in the *Curriculum Guidance for the Foundation Stage* (QCA). This document has paved the way for children's early learning to be followed through into Baseline Assessment measured on entry to school (from September 1998) and into National Curriculum assessment for school-age children. It was expected that the integration of these three would contribute to the earlier identification of children who were experiencing difficulties in making progress.

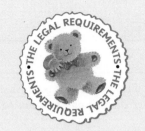

The Early Learning Goals have been set into context so that they are seen as an aid to planning ahead, rather than as an early years curriculum to replace 'learning through play'. Effective early years education needs both a relevant curriculum and practitioners who understand and are able to implement it. To this end, practical examples of Stepping Stones towards the Early Learning Goals are provided in the detailed curriculum guidance.

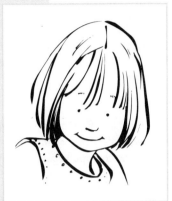

Within this book, each activity is linked to a learning objective for the entire group, and also linked to an individual learning target for any child who has speech and language difficulties. You will find that many of these individual targets relate to the area of Communication, language and literacy.

Degree of excellence

Defining a set of Early Learning Goals, which most children will have attained by the end of their Foundation Stage (the end of their Reception year), has helped to ensure that nursery education is of good quality and a sound preparation for later schooling. In order to make certain that nursery education is of a good standard, early years providers registered with their local Early Years Development and Childcare Partnership are required to have their educational provision inspected regularly. The nursery inspectors, appointed by the Office for Standards in Education (OFSTED), assess the quality of the early years educational provision and look at the clarity of roles and responsibilities within the setting. They are interested in plans for meeting the needs of individual children (including those with SEN) and developing improved partnerships with parents and carers.

Scottish framework

In Scotland, there is also a curriculum framework for three- to five-year-olds involving five key aspects of learning – Emotional, personal and social development (including Religious and moral development); Knowledge and understanding of the world (including Environmental studies and Mathematics); Communication and language; Expressive and aesthetic development, and Physical development and movement. The activities suggested within this book will also be relevant to these Areas of Learning.

The need for individual education plans

One characteristic of Early Years Action for a child with SEN is the writing of the individual education plan (IEP). This is a plan that aims to lead to the child making progress. An example of an IEP is shown on the next page with a photocopiable proforma on page 85. This plan should be reviewed regularly with parents and carers. It should be seen as an integrated aspect of the curriculum planning for the whole group and should only include that which is additional to or different from the differentiated early years curriculum which is in place for all the children. You may find the section on 'Differentiation' in the series handbook useful.

Individual education plan

Name: Ruben	**Stage:** 3

Nature of difficulty: Ruben has a difficulty in understanding abstract language and he speaks in short phrases that are not always clear. He also finds it hard to play socially with other children and he tends to lack confidence in new situations.

Action

1 Seeking further information
Davina will be Ruben's key worker. She will contact Ruben's speech and language therapist, Ms Turner, and see how the pre-school can work alongside her. She will set up a home/pre-school/therapist diary so that everyone can keep in touch over Ruben's targets and progress.

2 Seeking training
We would like to learn more about helping Ruben to develop his language skills, establish more appropriate ways of interacting with other children and feel more confident with other children. Jenny, our SENCO, will contact the early years partnership and the speech and language therapy service for information about any suitable training courses.

3 Assessing Ruben
We need a system of monitoring and recording Ruben's language and play that fits in with our pre-school activities. Davina will spend the first five sessions playing alongside Ruben so that he feels more confident. She will observe him as he plays, keeping running notes about the ways in which he has learned to interact with other children, examples of the words and phrases he uses, any words or phrases he did not seem to understand, and his strengths and interests.

4 Encouraging speech and language development
● We will plan activities around the abstract words that the therapist is teaching Ruben this term: long/short, heavy/light, full/empty, more/less.
● We will use Ruben's name and a light touch on the chin to ensure that he is looking at us and listening when we speak with him.
● We will speak to Ruben in clear and short phrases, emphasizing the key words.
● We will show Ruben what to do as well as tell him.
● We will echo back Ruben's phrases clearly to ensure that he both hears the clear version and that other children understand and respond to his speech.
● We will encourage interaction with other children by supporting Ruben in a small group of children for some of the activities.
● We will use music circle time for choosing activities to boost Ruben's language skills, self-esteem and confidence within the larger group.

Help from parents
Ruben's mum and dad, Madge and Jon, are soon to go on a Hanen training course. They have agreed to meet with the pre-school staff and share approaches. Madge will make a point of talking with Ruben's key worker, Davina, every Monday before pre-school and also to help to keep the home/pre-school/therapist diary up to date.

Targets for this term
● Ruben will play in the water tray for ten minutes and vocalize to the other children, supported by Davina. Ruben will 'show me' which of two objects or sets is long/short, heavy/light, full/empty, more/less with 90% accuracy.
● Ruben will begin to join in a favourite activity independently, playing alongside other children and occasionally speaking with them.
● Ruben will begin to look pleased when other children approach him and talk to him.
● Ruben will look at the speaker for at least three seconds when he is being spoken to.

Review meeting with parents
In six weeks' time. Invite the speech and language therapist, Ms Turner.

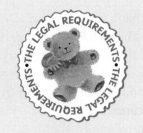

Working with parents and carers

Parents and carers often ask how they can help at home when areas of concern are expressed by staff in the early years setting. They might also approach you with their own concerns that they need you to address with them. Parents and carers are the primary educators of their children and should be included as an essential part of the whole-group approach to meeting a child's needs from the start. They have expert knowledge on their own children and you will need to create an ethos which shows how much this information is valued and made use of. Sharing information is important and is a two-way process.

The following are some practical ways of involving parents and carers in meeting their children's needs:

● Make a personal invitation to parents and carers. For various reasons, parents and carers do not always call into the setting on a daily basis. It is often helpful to invite them into your setting to share information about their children's achievements in an informal way, or, if possible, to arrange a home visit.

● Draw the parents and carers' attention to a specific display where examples of their children's work can be seen.

● Show parents and carers what their children have already achieved and improvements that have been made in their language development

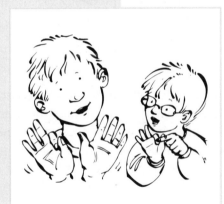

within the setting. Do not make them feel too despondent if there have not been improvements at home. Use the 'good news' as a hope for positive changes to come.

● Encourage the children to show their parents or carers what they can do or say, or what they have learned.

● Ask parents and carers for their opinions by allowing opportunities for them to contribute information and share experiences with you. It is often helpful to set a regular time aside when other demands will not intrude.

● Thank parents and carers regularly for their support.

● Celebrate success with parents and carers. This will ensure an ongoing positive partnership.

● Use the home/pre-school/therapist diary to keep in touch.

● A two- or three-way system of sharing information about a child's success, experiences and opportunities can help in supporting the child in each setting.

Working with outside agencies

When assessing and working with a young child who has SEN, an outside professional might be involved in helping staff to monitor and meet the child's needs. For children with speech and language difficulties, this is likely to be a speech and language therapist. Some children entering an early years setting may already be referred to a therapist or be on a waiting list for assessment. The kind of advice and support available will vary with local policies and practices.

Sometimes, a speech and language therapist might be involved in helping the child to make certain speech sounds more clearly, or to speak more fluently. It might be that, despite these difficulties, the child's speech can be clearly understood by you and by other children,

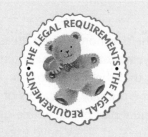

and that these difficulties do not affect the child's learning and communication in any way. You need not make an IEP for such children as they are not experiencing 'special educational needs' in any way. In other words, just because a speech and language therapist is delivering therapy, it does not follow that there are learning difficulties and that special procedures are needed within the setting.

However, if the speech and language therapy involves setting educational targets affecting the way that you interact with and teach that particular child, then you will need to take 'Early Years Action' and write out an IEP, preferably in conjunction with the therapist, and certainly liaising with the parents or carers.

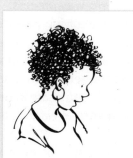

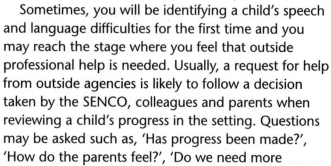

Sometimes, you will be identifying a child's speech and language difficulties for the first time and you may reach the stage where you feel that outside professional help is needed. Usually, a request for help from outside agencies is likely to follow a decision taken by the SENCO, colleagues and parents when reviewing a child's progress in the setting. Questions may be asked such as, 'Has progress been made?', 'How do the parents feel?', 'Do we need more information and advice on the child's needs from outside?' and so on. Referrals to the speech and language therapy service are usually made through the health service by contacting the school doctor or the health visitor.

Developing inclusive practice

'Inclusion' is the practice of including all the children together in a setting. The children participate fully in all the regular routines and activities of the classroom or playroom, though these might need to be modified to meet individual children's goals and objectives. The activities in this book carry both learning objectives for all the children (with and without SEN) and individual targets for the children who have SEN.

Factors that support inclusive practices

● Careful joint planning, especially to make sure that any within-class support is used effectively.

● The use of educational labels rather than categories or medical labels, such as 'language difficulty' rather than 'language disorder' or 'dysphasic', or even 'child who has SEN' rather than 'SEN child'.

● Teachers and adults who provide good role models for the children because of their positive expectations and the way that they respect and value the children.

● The use of strategies which improve the children's communication and behaviour.

● The use of teaching strategies which enable all the children to participate and learn.

● Individual approaches that draw on the children's earlier experiences, set high expectations and encourage mutual peer support.

● The flexible use of support aimed to promote joining in and inclusion rather than to create barriers and exclusion.

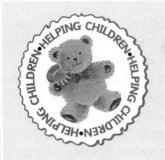

HELPING CHILDREN WITH SPEECH AND LANGUAGE DIFFICULTIES

This chapter gives an insight into why speech and language difficulties may arise, explains the different areas of language difficulties and gives suggestions on how to support children with these difficulties.

The activities covered in this book are suitable for a range of needs and difficulties. It is impossible to be prescriptive about a particular child in a setting, as each will have very individual needs, but this book enables you to dip into the suggestions and find those that seem to suit the particular special educational needs for your specific situation.

All of the activities include individual learning targets based on 'real' difficulties and involve approaches that have been found to be helpful in actual cases.

Speech or language difficulties

Speech and language difficulties may occur for different reasons. There might be a lack of opportunity for development because of deprivation or emotional causes, a hearing loss or physical disability, or a general difficulty in learning and development. Difficulties may arise even in the absence of these causes, being described as a 'specific developmental disorder of speech and language', 'language impairment' or 'specific language difficulty'.

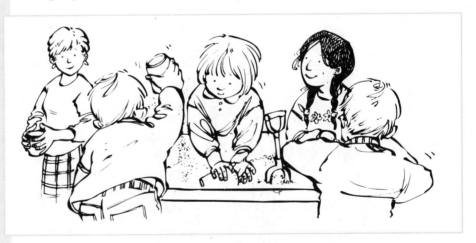

Children with speech and language difficulties may find it hard to speak clearly, express themselves using language or understand language, even though they can hear clearly and have had every opportunity to learn. These are the children 'targeted' in the activities in chapters three to eight of this book.

Another book in this series, *Sensory Difficulties*, gives ideas for supporting children who are slow to talk because of hearing impairment, though you may find some of the ideas in this book helpful, too. Some children have difficulties in communicating because English is not their first language. Although this book is not about these children, some of the activity ideas may be helpful.

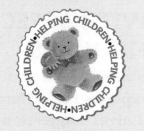

Children who do not speak clearly

Some situations involve children who do not speak distinctly and their language can only be understood by those who know them really well, and where there is a shared context so that the listener knows what the child is talking about. This might be because the child is slow to develop all of the speech sounds necessary to make clear speech, or perhaps they cannot co-ordinate the sounds in the required sequence. These children are sometimes described as having dyspraxic, dysarthric or articulation difficulties depending on the cause. They can quickly lose confidence if they cannot make themselves understood. They also lose heart if they are repeatedly asked to copy words clearly.

Speech and language therapy can help these children to learn and practise new sounds. It is helpful if settings link closely with any ongoing therapy so that activities can be planned around the therapy goals – for example, some children benefit from activities that help them hear the rhythm of syllables and language. Number rhymes and action rhymes are most beneficial. The use of symbols, pictures or real objects can be used when the child is asked to make a choice or to plan their session. Hearing back the correct enunciation of a word, without being asked to repeat it, can provide the child with the correct model of the word and also help the listener to clarify what the child was trying to say. Patient listening and interpretation is called for, with plenty of opportunities for the child to succeed in areas of play that do not involve language.

If the speech is very unclear, the speech and language therapist might recommend that these children be taught to use a simple sign

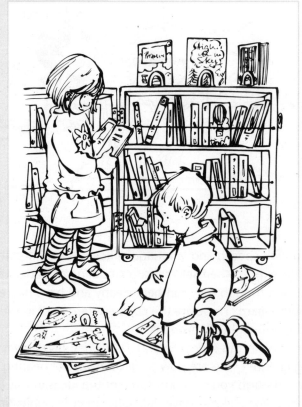

language such as 'Makaton' (see page 96). This is not used to replace their speech but used to help other people understand the words that they are trying to communicate so that they can respond appropriately.

Delayed language development

For other children, language remains shortened like a telegram because they do not naturally acquire the grammar and order that language usually follows. Sometimes this is because their language development is delayed, but nevertheless progressing along normal lines. Perhaps these children are delayed in other areas of their development as well and the language delay is just one part of this immaturity. Activities which help the child progress step by small step will be the most helpful, making sure that the child has a chance to succeed and develop confidence at each stage. You will find more ideas in *Learning Difficulties* which is another book in this series.

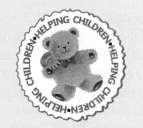

Specific language disorder or difficulty

For those children with specific language disorder or difficulty, their understanding of language, and especially abstract language such as 'big', 'empty' and other concept words, is usually affected as well as their use of language. You might hear these children described as having difficulties in language 'expression' (speaking) and/or 'comprehension' or 'reception' (listening and understanding).

Expressive language difficulties

Children with expressive language difficulties might use very short phrases or have difficulties in remembering the names of things. They

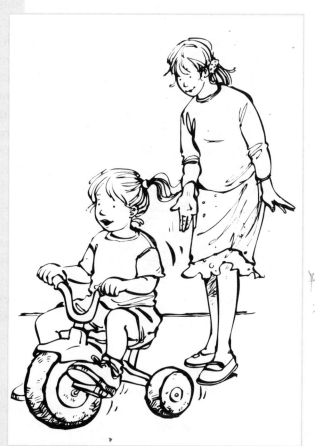

might use general descriptions such as 'thing' rather than the label. Their speech might sound 'babyish' even though they have developed age-appropriate skills in other areas. Some tend to lose fluency when they are excited or stressed, and talk best in a relaxed situation. Some children stutter and this becomes worse if they feel pressured or if attention is drawn to it.

Again, it is helpful for these children to hear correct models of what they are trying to say, for example, repeat back 'Yes, *James* is riding the *bike*' to the child's 'James bike'. It is also helpful for them to be given choices or alternatives when being asked a question such as, 'Do you want to play in the *house* or on the *bike*?'. Picture books and concrete props during story time can help the development of vocabulary. When the child is trying to remember a word, you can help by suggesting other clues such as, 'What did it look like?' and 'What was it for?' to help the child develop descriptions.

Comprehension or receptive language difficulties

This disorder can be difficult to detect. You might think that the child understands everything you say, yet on close examination you find that they are responding to a host of other clues rather than to the words alone. Test this out by offering no clues: 'Put your coat on' might well gain a response at the end of the session when everyone is getting ready to go home, but would it gain the same response if you said it in the middle of the session?

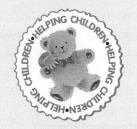

Observation diaries can be a useful way of keeping a track of words and phrases that the child seemed to find difficult to understand. You can model ways of speaking and playing that the child can then learn from. Link actions, pictures or real objects to concept words such as 'heavy' or 'high' so that the child eventually learns what they mean. You can then help them to generalize what they have learned to new situations and new activities. These children may find it difficult to transfer what they have learned from one situation to another because they can be rather rigid and unimaginative in their play.

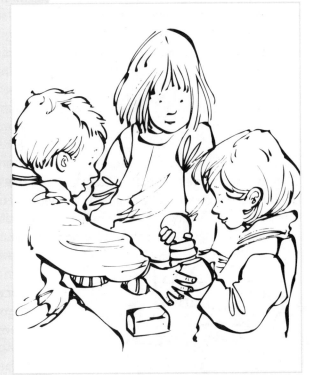

Pragmatic difficulties

Quite often, children who have specific language difficulties also have difficulties in understanding social situations, seeing the other point of view, using their imaginations and handling conversations. Social skills can be modelled and taught, with sharing and turn-taking games used to support this.

Many of the activities in this book also aim to improve the children's pragmatic skills. Another book in the series, *Autistic Spectrum Difficulties*, gives more ideas on helping children with pragmatic difficulties.

The prevalence and causes

Because of the differences between professionals in how they define the population of children with specific speech and language difficulties, it is difficult to be precise about prevalence. Studies have suggested pre-school prevalence rates from three to 15 per cent of the population. It appears that some children overcome an initial delay fairly early on, but others go on to experience later language and literacy difficulties if their early problems are not resolved. In one study, 60 per cent of children who had language difficulties during their pre-school years continued to exhibit language problems at the age of ten and even beyond. Nevertheless, about 40 per cent of children who had language difficulties at the age of four had resolved these problems by the middle of their fifth years. The prognosis was poorest for those who had general learning difficulties as well.

This makes the years leading up to the compulsory full-time schooling a particularly vital time for intervention. In this book, you will find suggestions for planning activities which help all the children to work towards the Early Learning Goals, but which are also individually targeted for any child who might have any one of a range of speech and language difficulties. You will need to select and choose approaches,

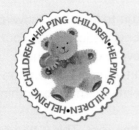

and not just activities, to suit your situation. In order to do this, it is helpful to understand the general teaching approaches which have proved effective when working with young children who have speech and language difficulties.

Making observations

Do you have children with these needs in your setting?
- Some children still need help to speak clearly.
- Some children have a very limited vocabulary.
- Some children can only speak in very short phrases.
- Some children can only understand very simple language and instructions.
- Some children cannot grasp the meaning of abstract language.
- Some children cannot use language imaginatively or in conversations.
- Some children do not understand what is yet expected of them in social situations.

Educational implications

Talking is such a central part of early learning that you will find it more difficult to gauge what the child has learned and understood and to build on their learning. The best help that you can give the child will be your own language, but delivered at just the right level of complexity or

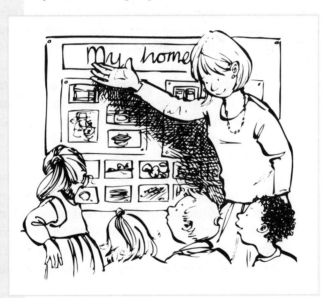

simplicity for the child to understand it. This means that you need to get to know the child well. Talk with the parents or carers and find out about how much the child understands and how well they can express themselves. How do they make their needs known? Ask parents to tape some language at home, where the child is most relaxed, so that you can have a 'feel' of their stage of development even if the child says very little in the setting. Get in touch with the speech and language therapist to share assessments and targets. It is easier to understand what the child is trying to tell you if you are talking about things you have done or shared together. Use props and photographs from home to trigger talk about the child's 'news'. Use picture books and real objects to introduce topics. Start with subjects that really interest the child.

In the early stages, talk will relate to everyday objects, names and activities in the 'here and now'. Introduce words for toys, actions, smells, colours and textures as you introduce new experiences. Comment on the child's play to show your interest and to provide

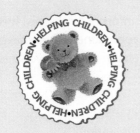

models for them. Some children find it difficult to learn the 'flow' of speaking first, then listening. Support free conversations by encouraging simple turn-taking and teach the children how to gain attention appropriately with an 'excuse me' rather than a direct interruption. Keep your conversations simple and try to relate them to something you all know about at first.

It is tempting to bombard children with questions. This is particularly demanding for many children with language difficulties as they do not understand the meaning of the question words such as 'what' or 'why'. This is one of the reasons why they might tend to echo what you have said rather than answer it, or give you an answer that simply does not fit. Instead, provide simple commentaries about what the child is doing and offer choices where possible, for example, 'Do you want the *red* one or the *blue* one?'.

Looking for special opportunities

How can adults in early years settings support children who have speech and language difficulties? The following suggestions come from research carried out for I CAN, the national educational charity for children with speech and language difficulties (see page 96).

● Try to interpret the child's needs

For a child who is having difficulty in making their needs known, appoint a key worker to get to know that child well and to find out about the way that they communicate and make their needs known. This key worker will then be able to interpret the child's actions and act on them consistently, thereby ensuring any signalling of need becomes meaningful and intentional. They can also put together a 'communication book', with photographs and descriptions, showing all staff the signs, expressions, words or behaviours that the child uses in order to communicate their feelings and needs.

The key worker can also come to know the child well enough to know when to stop the questioning and all the input and allow the child space. Children who have speech and language difficulties can quickly feel 'overloaded' if there is too much noise, language or too many expectations upon then. When you realize that it is time to stop, have some calming activities on hand such as playing with the train set, or lying on cushions in the book corner with soothing music to help the child wind down.

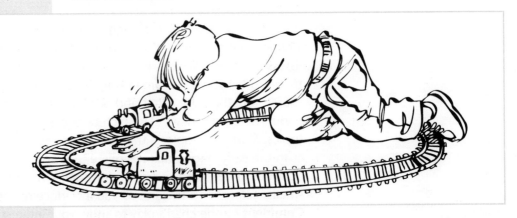

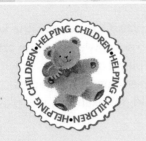

● Provide a simple commentary about what the child is doing

Play alongside the child with speech and language difficulties and provide a simple spoken commentary of the child's play. This provides opportunities for the child to link action with word and can also help other children to interpret what the child is doing and saying. Keep your language simple and at the child's level of understanding, emphasizing key words appropriately.

Encourage the child with disordered language to describe things in an organized way by keeping your commentary well structured. Ask questions such as, 'Who was involved?', 'Where are they?', 'What are they doing?', 'What happened next?' and so on.

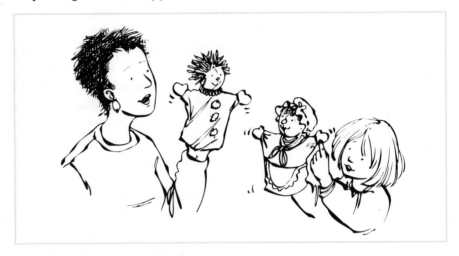

● Use non-verbal modelling to give the child more information

For a child with a limited repertoire of play, you can model and extend their play. They can be shown, as well as told, how to stack the bricks, play with the puppets and match the animals. Children with speech and language difficulties sometimes have problems with fine motor co-ordination and you may need to show them how to use a pencil or paintbrush, how to enjoy mark-making and drawing and how to dress and undress. Breaking these skills down into fine steps so that each step is possible, and achievable, is the best way forward. Praise the child for each effort, gradually building up their confidence.

● Teach the child to play reciprocally

Encourage the development of reciprocal play for a child who lacks the skills of social turn-taking. This important skill leads on to language and conversation later. Simple 'my turn, your turn' activities and games help the development of this skill. Start by playing together with the same toy so that the child learns to share the toy with one other adult who nevertheless keeps the game fun. Then move on to definite turn-taking games and early conversations. Blow bubbles for the child to burst, roll a large ball between you, use puppets and toy telephones to encourage a spoken reaction.

● Facilitate the child's joining in

Use your presence, suggestions and support to make it easier for a child with communication difficulties to join in with other children. Sometimes the key worker might have to interpret what the child is

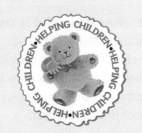

saying to their peers in order to sustain the play. Occasionally, the key worker may prompt and support the child in acknowledging the other children's presence and contribution to the play. Look for ways of making the social play more enjoyable for everyone; some games can only be played if there is more than one child, for example, ball play or pushing a truck that has another child in it.

● Support turn-taking and sharing
Consistently encourage turn-taking and sharing for a child who would find these skills particularly difficult. Games such as *Snap*, *Lotto*, *Pairs* and *Snakes and ladders* have all proved helpful. They also provide opportunities for recognizing, talking about and resolving feelings.

● Support and encourage receptive language skills
Provide language at just the right level for a child with language difficulties to understand and respond to. Use and emphasize just one or two simple key words that you know the child can understand. Perhaps rephrase instructions that have been given to the whole group, keeping them concrete and showing the child what to do as well. When you are sharing books together, spend time discussing the pictures and predicting what might happen next. Encourage the child to retell the story in their own way, gradually building up to longer sequences. Perhaps at first, for example, a child might predict what is beneath the flap in a familiar 'lift-the-flap' book. In time, they may tell you a whole section of the story and remember what happens at the end of the story as well.

● Provide continual reassurance
Provide a higher level of reassurance, just by staying close or by watching on. A child with speech and language difficulties is more likely to lack confidence and feel insecure in a social setting, and may even find the company of other children threatening. This is because they are not sure what to do or how to say things. They might find other children unpredictable or frightening because they have not learned the simple rules of social behaviour. They are likely to feel more confident if you are close by to encourage and reassure them.

● Teach social skills
Encourage appropriate social skills and behaviour for a child likely to be experiencing difficulties in understanding social situations. These children may have to be taught social skills directly that other children

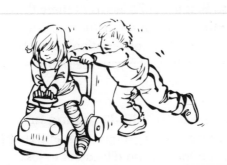

might pick up naturally. This is not because they are 'naughty', although they often get described as such.

By getting to know the child well, and by trying to see the world from their point of view, you will be able to adopt more flexible ways of supporting and teaching them. The child might

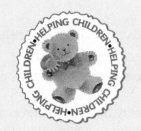

need to learn how to make their voice loud or soft when talking and not to shout or whisper all the time. They may need to learn to look at you when speaking and how close to stand. They might need to be shown how to be 'gentle', how to greet other children without being too shy or too overwhelming, how to pass a toy to another child rather than throwing it, or how to ask for a toy rather than to grab it. Identify which behaviour you need to change and decide what new behaviour needs to be taught in its place.

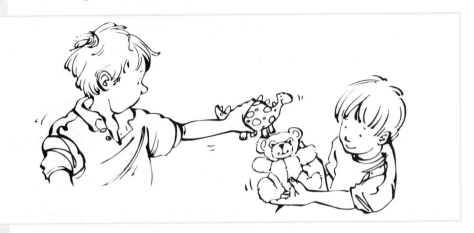

● Assist the development of pragmatic skills

Some children have pragmatic difficulties in using language and communication in a social context. They find it hard to see another person's point of view and can appear to be antisocial or socially withdrawn. Where a child has pragmatic difficulties, help them to see another child's point of view and maintain a flow to their interaction.

Encourage early conversations where one of you speaks and the other listens. Invite eye contact by using the child's name, a gentle touch on the shoulder and by speaking at their level, face to face. Praise them for looking at you when you speak to them and also encourage them to look at you when they are speaking to you. Help the child to stay on the subject if they tend to wander. Gently point out that you need to listen to the other children too, using a gentle hand-hold to show that you are still 'there' for them while they wait for their turn to speak.

● Support the child during large group play

Assist the child when they are playing within a large group of other children whose language skills are more proficient. Children whose speech and language development is progressing normally are excellent models for children who have difficulties. Draw attention to the other children's questions and comments and support the child with difficulties in responding, playing co-operatively or initiating ideas themselves. Start in a small group of two children and gradually extend the size of the group, step by step.

Many of the activities in this book are suggested as suitable for small groups, but you may find that you can have larger groups of children once progress has been made. Above all, do expect progress: you are planning inclusive activities not just because the child has special needs, but because you are actually going to meet those needs and see progress.

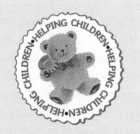

● Extend the child's imaginative play

Help the child to play imaginatively and develop symbolic skills. This is especially helpful if the child can learn to play imaginatively with another child, providing opportunities for developing their own imaginative ideas and language.

Encourage imaginative play and pretend play by basing this on 'real life' experiences at first. You might act out going to a party together or visiting the supermarket. Miniature play such as with small-world construction toys can also be helpful and will mean that other children enjoy playing as well. You can also use puppets and real props to illustrate stories and talk-about sessions, making these more concrete and accessible for the child who has speech and language difficulties.

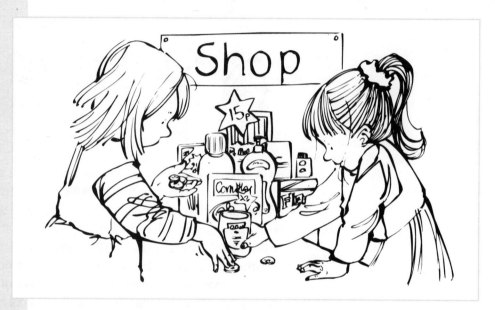

● Support the child's expressive language

Encourage the child to speak and communicate with others more proficient than themselves, thereby benefiting from both their models and their responses. If speech is unclear or brief, repeat back what the child has said clearly and in its fuller form. Emphasize the key words clearly, taking care not to 'overload' the child with language way beyond their ability, for example:

Child: Jack car!

Adult: Yes, *Jack* has the *car*. Would *you* like a turn?

● Support the child's planning and persistence

Help the child to plan what they are going to do next and encourage them to see this through and evaluate how it has gone and what they think about it.

Spend time at the beginning of an activity talking with the child about what you are going to do together and how – for example, if you are about to make a sandwich together, talk about different kinds of fillings, focus on how you will make the sandwich and then on how you will serve or eat it. It can be helpful and reassuring to a child who has language difficulties if you use pictures or symbols to help them understand the sequence of events during their session.

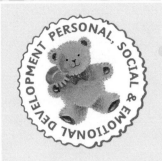

PERSONAL, SOCIAL AND EMOTIONAL DEVELOPMENT

This chapter encourages all the children's personal, social and emotional development as well as targeting particular speech and language skills in children who have difficulties.

PERSONAL, SOCIAL & EMOTIONAL DEVELOPMENT

In the bag

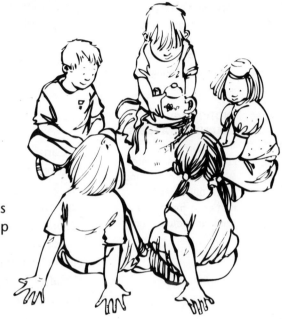

Group size
Six to eight children

What you need
A dark-coloured cloth drawstring bag; box; selection of three or four related objects with distinctive shapes, such as a plastic teapot, plate, cup and spoon, or a tambourine, shaker, bells and triangle.

What to do
Choose sets of objects that relate to a particular activity or topic as a way of introducing the children to any new vocabulary.

Ask the children to sit in a circle. Show them the items and then pass them around the circle. Invite individual children to name them. Ask the group to think of different ways in which all of your objects link together, such as 'in the play house' or 'at music time'.

Now place all the items in the bag. Invite a child to find the teapot just by feeling the shapes in the bag. Let them pull it out. Were they correct? If not, remove that item and let the child have another turn until they succeed. Celebrate this success. Now replace all the items in the bag and ask the next child to find something else.

When everyone has had a turn, hide the items in a box and secretly place just one item in the bag. Pass it to the first child. Can they tell you what it is? Lift it out and have a look. Were they correct? Place a different item in the bag for the next child's turn.

Special support
Make sure that the child that you are targeting knows the names of the objects. If necessary, teach them individually before the activity.

Extension
Let the children take turns to place an item in the bag for the next child to guess. Play a yes/no feely game, for example, 'Is it a teapot?', 'Is it the triangle?' and so on.

LEARNING OBJECTIVE FOR ALL THE CHILDREN
● to maintain attention, concentration and sit quietly when appropriate.

INDIVIDUAL LEARNING TARGET
● to identify a familiar object when given its name.

LINKS WITH HOME
Send a picture sheet home for parents and carers to help their children to learn any new vocabulary associated with a new topic such as 'On the farm' or 'At the zoo'. Suggest useful picture books that their children could borrow from the library ready for any new topic, particularly where the children may have difficulties in remembering the new words.

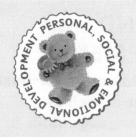

Good morning!

Group size
Whole group.

What you need
Just the children.

What to do
Familiarize yourself with the welcome song below. Sing it to the tune of 'Polly Wolly Doodle' (Traditional).

> Good morning *(child's name)*! Good morning *(child's name)*!
> And how are you today?
> It's good to see you here again
> So have a lovely play!

Carry out this activity at the beginning of the session. Invite the children to sit in a circle, then sing the song and move around the inside of the circle, facing each child in turn. Encourage them to give you eye contact and a smile in the first line, shake your hand in the second line and give you a wave in the third.

As the children become familiar with the song, pause before saying each child' name, encouraging them to add it in. If you are meeting in the afternoon, you can substitute 'Good morning (child's name)!' with 'Good afternoon (child's name)!' or 'Hello (child's name)!' as you prefer.

Special support
Children who have pragmatic difficulties as well as a speech and language difficulties often find it hard to give eye contact. Use a light touch and make sure that you are at their level in order to encourage the briefest of eye contacts as you sing to them. If the child that you are targeting uses Makaton sign language, you can use the greeting 'Good' (right thumb up) 'Morning' (fold your right arm across the front of your body and then draw your fist back across your body as if drawing the curtains aside).

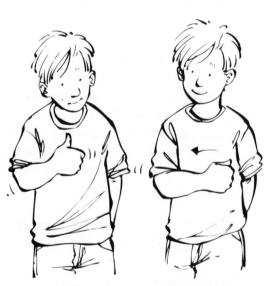

Good   **Morning**

Extension
Invite older children to help you greet the other children.

LEARNING OBJECTIVE FOR ALL THE CHILDREN
● to be confident to try new activities, initiate ideas and speak in a familiar group.

INDIVIDUAL LEARNING TARGETS
● to give eye contact when greeted
● to wave a greeting
● to give their names in front of a familiar group.

LINKS WITH HOME
Encourage the parents or carers of the child that you are targeting to say their child's name and establish eye contact before giving them simple instructions or greeting them.

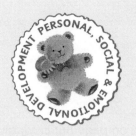

LEARNING OBJECTIVE FOR ALL THE CHILDREN
● to be confident to try new activities.

INDIVIDUAL LEARNING TARGET
● to join in with key sounds.

Monster rap

Group size
Eight to ten children.

What you need
Just the children.

What to do
Teach the children the rap below. Stamp your feet and swing your arms as you chant it together.

> Monsters in the jungle,
> Circling around;
> Growling at their friends and
> Clawing at the ground;
> Listen to their voices
> What an eerie sound!
> OO – AA – OO – AA!
> *OO – AA – OO – AA!*
>
> *Hannah Mortimer*

Invent other sounds that the monsters could make and try them together. Raise your arms as you make the sounds. Stay close to any children who might be anxious, or let them watch until they feel ready to join in.

Special support
This rhyme provides a simple repetitive sound to practise repeated vowel sounds. Have a practice together first and exaggerate your own mouth movements to help the children form the sounds clearly. Keep the activity fun so that the child that you are targeting wants to join in, rather then feels pressured to.

Extension
Encourage the children to help you make up another verse to the rap together with new actions and sounds.

LINKS WITH HOME
If the child that you are targeting has difficulties in speaking clearly, find out from the parents or carers which speech sounds they are working on at the moment (probably with the speech and language therapist). Try to think of a suitable monster sound to reinforce this and send your rhyme home for the child to practise and have fun with.

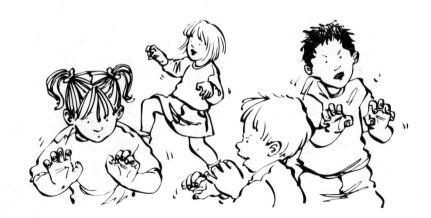

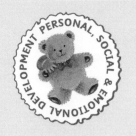

LEARNING OBJECTIVE FOR ALL THE CHILDREN
● to have a developing awareness of their own feelings.

INDIVIDUAL LEARNING TARGET
● to link words with expressions and feelings.

Smiles and frowns

Group size
Four to six children

What you need
A hand-held mirror; the photocopiable sheet on page 86; card; glue.

What to do
Make an enlarged copy of the photocopiable sheet. Cut out the four faces and mount these onto separate pieces of card. Sit in a circle with the children and show them the picture of a happy face. Ask, 'Who can make a happy face?'. Choose a child and say, 'Daniel looks really happy! Can you all make a face like Daniel?'. Ask the children what makes them happy and what they enjoy doing when they are happy. Repeat for the other expressions on the cards.

Follow on the activity by whispering to one child and suggesting that they make a sad face. Invite the other children to tell you what kind of face the child has made and then to copy it. Repeat for the other three expressions.

Special support
Children with language difficulties will find your questioning hard to understand. Accept any ideas that the child that you are targeting gives you that are associated with happy, sad, angry or scared feelings. If necessary, help them to recognize the expression by looking at the features. Say, 'Look! She's smiling so she must be happy'.

Extension
Help the children to make their own drawings of happy, sad, angry and scared faces to use in this game.

LINKS WITH HOME
Tell parents and carers which 'feeling' words you have been discussing in your setting, and ask them to talk with their children about things that make them feel happy, sad, angry and scared at home.

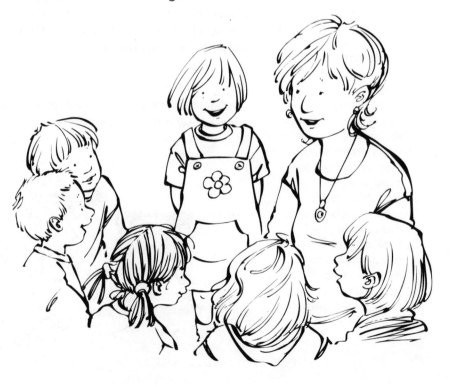

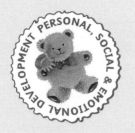

LEARNING OBJECTIVE FOR ALL THE CHILDREN
● to maintain attention while listening.

INDIVIDUAL LEARNING TARGET
● to remember and repeat two spoken words.

Red lorry, yellow lorry

Group size
Four to six children.

What you need
A small plastic bucket; 'magic wand' or glittery stick; selection of small treats such as jelly bears or stickers.

What to do
Gather the children together and talk about words. Which words do the children enjoy saying? Tell some nursery rhymes together with phrases such as 'Georgie Porgie, Pudding and Pie'. Share some tongue-twisters with the children, such as those in *The Oxford Nursery Rhyme Book* assembled by Iona and Peter Opie (OUP), including:

Swan swam over the sea,
Swim, swan, swim!
Swan swam back again,
Well swum swan!
(Traditional)

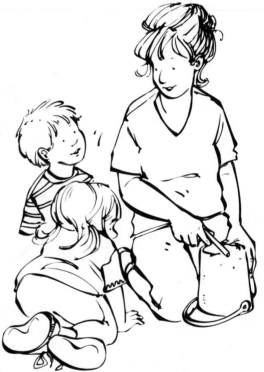

Now suggest to the children that you play a game with words. Hide the treats about your person so that you can put one underneath the upturned bucket without the children seeing. Tap your 'magic wand' onto the bucket and say the tongue-twister. If the children tell you that you said it correctly, lift up the bucket. If you have said it correctly, you will have put a treat underneath, if not, you will not have hidden any. Let each child have a turn and decide together what 'magic words' the child should say, for example, 'Red brick, blue brick, red brick, blue brick' or 'Flibberty-gibberty-flibberty-pop!', depending on their ability and their own ideas. Make sure that everybody 'wins' a treat!

Special support
Choose two words or sounds that are at the correct level for the child that you are targeting. If they cannot say them clearly, model the correct response but still allow their reward.

Extension
Tell the children the tongue-twisters 'Red lorry, yellow lorry, red lorry, yellow lorry' and 'She sells sea shells on the sea-shore'. Encourage them to repeat these as quickly as they can.

LINKS WITH HOME
If a child is learning how to speak clearly, perhaps because they have immature speech sounds or they have verbal dyspraxia, ask the parents or carers to carry a notebook between the speech and language therapist, home and your setting so that you can build on their child's learning.

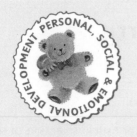

Row the boat

Group size
Ten to 20 children.

What you need
Just the children.

What to do
Sit on the floor with the children and encourage each child to find a partner. Help them to sit opposite each other so that they can hold hands and rock forwards and backwards. Sing the following rhyme as you rock:

> Row, row, row your boat,
> Gently down the stream;
> Merrily, merrily, merrily, merrily,
> Life is but a dream!
> (Traditional)

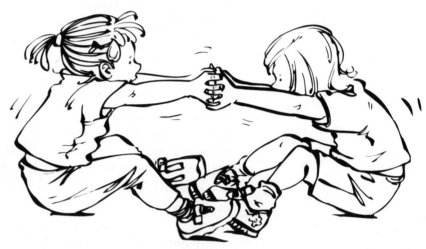

Now introduce some new versions for the last two lines, for example, 'If you see a big baboon, don't forget to swoon!' (everybody falls over to the 'ooooo' sound); 'If you see a prowling lion, don't forget to scream!' (everybody screams) and 'If you see a hippopotamus, don't forget to make a lot of fuss!' (everybody cries).

You can invent many more together; it does not matter if they do not rhyme, so long as they help to practise many different sounds.

End with a final verse of the traditional rhyme again.

Special support
Rehearse some of the sounds together before you begin the activity, or encourage the child that you are targeting to think of some animal noises themselves which you can build into the song. Let the child experiment with non-speech sounds in order for them to gain confidence. Stay close to the child (but do not partner yourself) so that you can encourage them.

Extension
Invite the children to think of a new verse for the rhyme.

LEARNING OBJECTIVE FOR ALL THE CHILDREN
● to work as part of a group.

INDIVIDUAL LEARNING TARGET
● to experiment with voice sounds.

LINKS WITH HOME
Ask parents and carers to share an animal picture book with their children and to practise animal sounds together.

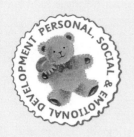

LEARNING OBJECTIVE FOR ALL THE CHILDREN
● to form good relationships with adults and peers.

INDIVIDUAL LEARNING TARGET
● to develop early conversational skills.

Ring-a-ling

Group size
Eight to ten children.

What you need
Two toy telephones; a large glove puppet, for example, 'Molly' available from LDA (see page 96).

What to do
Sit in a circle with the children and introduce your glove puppet. Explain that the puppet is very shy and does not like to use the telephone. Encourage the children to tell it what to do. Make the puppet pick up the receiver of one of the toy telephones and dial a number. Then say to a child, 'It's for you!'. Ask the child to lift the receiver of the other telephone as the puppet says, rather tentatively, 'Hello? Who's there?'. Encourage the child to say their name. The puppet then asks, 'Will you be my friend?' to which the child replies and then says 'Goodbye'. You can develop the conversations as the activity progresses, making sure that the puppet telephones each child.

Let each child telephone the puppet in turn and ask a question or hold a simple conversation. Praise the children for making the puppet feel so welcome.

Special support
Sit beside the child that you are targeting and keep the conversation simple, encouraging them to say their name and listen between bouts of speaking. Some children with language difficulties find it hard to stop speaking long enough to allow the listener to reply, so this needs to be supported and encouraged.

Extension
Let the children use toy or unused 'real' telephones in the role-play area. Encourage simple conversations as part of a game of 'Offices' or 'Doctor's surgery'.

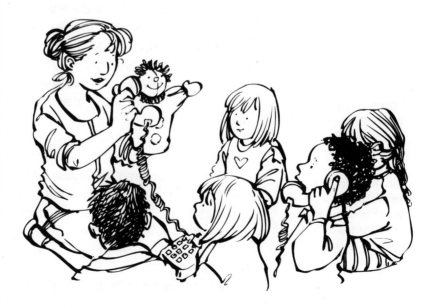

LINKS WITH HOME
Ask parents and carers to find an opportunity for their children to develop real telephone conversations with a favourite relative or friend.

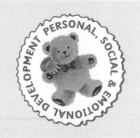

PERSONAL, SOCIAL & EMOTIONAL DEVELOPMENT

LEARNING OBJECTIVE FOR ALL THE CHILDREN
● to understand that people have different needs and views.

INDIVIDUAL LEARNING TARGET
● to see the other person's point of view.

Nid and Nod

Group size
Six to eight children.

What you need
Two glove puppets; small toy; biscuit; small stick.

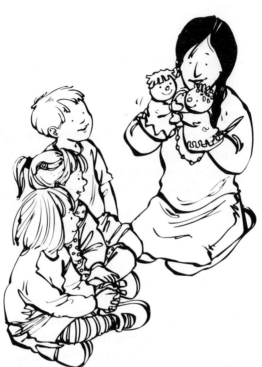

What to do
Gather the children together and introduce your two puppets as 'Nid' and 'Nod'. Tell the children a story in which Nid was playing happily one day with his favourite toy when Nod came and snatched the toy away. Mime Nod playing with the toy while Nid is crying. Ask the children what they think will happen now. Talk about how sad Nid feels and why. What should Nod do? Follow the children's suggestions as Nod gives the toy back, comforts Nid and they play together happily.

Now tell another story in which Nod was eating her biscuit at snack time when along came Nid and snatched the biscuit away. Mime Nod being cross and fighting with Nid, punching him and hitting him. Now both puppets are crying! Ask the children what they think will happen now. Talk this through as the puppets make up and share the biscuit together.

Tell the children that Nod is playing happily when Nid decides to play a fighting game. Nid rushes past Nod and hits her on the head with his stick. How does Nod feel now? Again talk this through together and try to resolve it.

Follow the activity up by looking at real examples of children being upset. Remind the group of their ideas about making one another feel better again.

Special support
Children with pragmatic language difficulties find it particularly hard to understand how another child might be thinking. Use this kind of puppet play to enable you to talk about feelings with the child that you are targeting or in a very small group.

Extension
Encourage the children to act out the stories using small-world toys.

LINKS WITH HOME
When the child that you are targeting does something antisocial at home, ask the parents or carers to encourage the child to tell them in simple words how they are feeling and why.

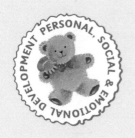

Now you see it

Group size
Four to six children.

What you need
A tray; box; six pairs of objects which differ in one respect, for example, a red brick and a blue brick, a big tractor and a little tractor, a full plastic bottle of cola and an empty bottle of cola, a heavy plastic jar and a light plastic jar and so on.

What to do
Place the pairs of items into a box. Sit in a circle with the children and show them all the objects, placing them on the tray and sharing words to describe them together. Emphasize the describing words such as 'red', 'blue', 'full', 'empty' and so on. Explain to the children that you are going to choose just six to show them. Select three of the pairs of objects and invite the children to look at them for approximately ten seconds. Now tell them that you will hide one and they have to tell you which one is missing.

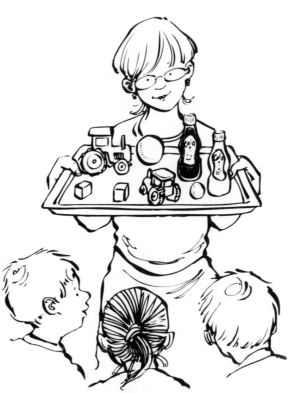

Remove the tray to one side and secretly take one of the items away, hiding it in your box. Can the children guess what is missing? Encourage them to use their describing words to name the missing item. Draw it out of the box for them to see if they were correct. Repeat for three more sets of items.

Special support
Start with fewer pairs of items. Some children with language difficulties have problems with remembering abstract concepts such as 'heavy', 'light', 'big', 'small' and so on. Offer a choice, for example, 'Is it the big one or the small one?'. If the child that you are targeting has difficulty in finding words from their vocabulary, provide the first sound to help them, such as 'It's r...' (red).

Extension
Extend the number of items and introduce more categories such as 'the big, red tractor' or 'the little blue one'.

LEARNING OBJECTIVE FOR ALL THE CHILDREN
● to maintain attention while looking.

INDIVIDUAL LEARNING TARGET
● to use describing words.

LINKS WITH HOME
Keep a note of concepts that are particularly difficult for the child that you are targeting to identify such as 'long' or 'short'. Send a task home for the parents or carers to teach and practise, such as 'Give me the long one' or 'Point to the short one'. Let the child take home a copy of the photocopiable sheet on page 87 to play with their parents or carers.

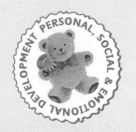

Play time

Group size
Whole group.

What you need
Just the children.

What to do
Sing this song at the end of circle time or music time as a transition between group time and play time, or group time and another activity. Adapt the words to suit your situation. The song is sung to the tune of 'Girls and Boys Come Out to Play' (Traditional):

> Now it's the end of circle time
> *(say two of the children's names)*
> If you want to go and play, that's fine!
>
> *Sinnington Playgroup*

At the end of the first line, pause to select two children's names, and encourage them to respond by leaving the circle and moving on to their next activity.

Repeat the song until all the children have moved away. If you are left with an odd number of children towards the end, say three children's names for the final verse so that no child is left behind.

Special support
Some children with language difficulties find the transition between one activity and another particularly difficult, especially if they are not sure about what is expected of them. The fact that you are selecting children in pairs will give the child that you are targeting the extra confidence to respond to their name. They can also gain

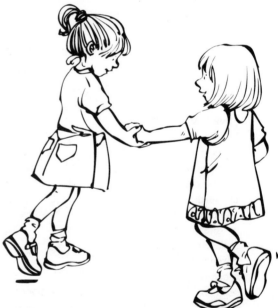

clues as to what is expected from them by watching their partner. Encourage their eye contact as you say their name and make sure that they are clear about what activity they are moving on to next.

Extension
Pause at the end of the verse to ask the children what they are going to do next, giving them choices if necessary. Help them to plan ahead.

LEARNING OBJECTIVE FOR ALL THE CHILDREN
● to be confident to speak in a familiar group.

INDIVIDUAL LEARNING TARGETS
● to wave or say 'Goodbye'
● to give eye contact.

LINKS WITH HOME
Use a version of the song above at the end of the session when parents and carers arrive. Explain to the parents or carers of the child that you are targeting that you are trying to encourage the child to use eye contact when saying 'Hello' and 'Goodbye'.

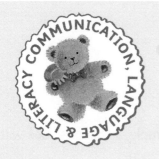

COMMUNICATION, LANGUAGE AND LITERACY

This chapter will help all the children to develop confidence in communication, language and literacy. There are special pointers for supporting children who may find this area particularly difficult.

LEARNING OBJECTIVES FOR ALL THE CHILDREN
● to explore and experiment with sounds
● to link sounds with letters.

INDIVIDUAL LEARNING TARGET
● to practise saying speech sounds.

LINKS WITH HOME
Let each child take home a copy of the photocopiable sheet and invite them to colour the pictures and point out the letters to their parents or carers. Ask the parents or carers of the child that you are targeting to practise the sounds at home.

Buzzy bee

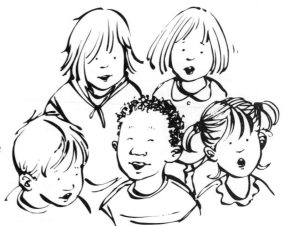

Group size
Six to eight children.

What you need
The photocopiable sheet on page 88; a series of cards, each showing the letter sounds that you are going to practise, for example, 'z', 'b', 'm', 'l' and 's'.

What to do
Gather the children around and teach them 'The buzzy bee song' on the photocopiable sheet to the tune of 'Twinkle, Twinkle, Little Star'. Sing the sounds slowly. (You can adapt the song to suit most sounds that you wish to practise.) While all the children may be practising linking written letter to spoken sound, any child that you are targeting will be able to rehearse certain specific speech sounds. Do not be afraid to use your imagination! You might add, for example, 'Grandad's gone and hurt his toe… a-a-a' or 'Watch the engine puffing home… f-f-f' or even 'Mummy's trying to start her car… g-g-g' and so on.

As you sing each verse, hold up the card showing the appropriate letter sound. Once the children are familiar with the song, place the letter cards on the floor and invite them to select the correct letter as you sing. As the children become more confident, hold up a letter card, ask them what sound it makes and then sing the verse that goes with that sound.

Special support
If the child that you are targeting has enunciation problems, use a home/pre-school/therapist diary to keep up to date with which speech sounds the therapist wishes the child to practise. Use this activity in a one-to-one situation, or in a very small group, to practise the sounds before you sing the song in a larger group. Give special and personal praise to a child who is trying especially hard to say the sounds clearly.

Extension
Encourage the children to trace over the letter cards, and invite each child to illustrate their letter with a train, cow or whatever matches the letter that they have chosen.

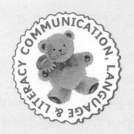

Echo box

Group size
Four to six children.

What you need
A quiet area; small decorated box, for example, a chocolate box with a flapped or hinged lid.

What to do
Sit in a circle with the children and ask them if they know what an echo is. Invite them to echo your sounds as you use a singsong voice. Call 'cuc-koo' and encourage the children to echo the sound. Go around the circle calling each child's name and invite everyone to echo it back.

Now show the children the decorated box. Pretend that it is a special echo box. Lift the lid, say a word loudly and clearly into the box such as 'cuc-koo', then shut the flap quickly. Share your enjoyment as you ask the children whether they are ready for you to let the sound out of the box. Lift the flap and repeat 'cuc-koo' as you pretend that the sound is flying out. Go around the circle inviting each child to put a sound into the box. Close the flap as soon as they have put their sound in, then encourage everyone to echo that sound as you raise the flap again.

Finally, put a sound into the box and invite individual children to lift the flap and 'let the sound out', repeating what you have said.

Special support
Make sure that the sound that you ask the child that you are targeting to repeat is within their repertoire.

Extension
Let the children record short phrases on a tape recorder and listen to their voices.

LEARNING OBJECTIVE FOR ALL THE CHILDREN
● to enjoy using spoken language to sustain attentive listening.

INDIVIDUAL LEARNING TARGETS
● to repeat back a word or short phrase
● to hear their own words repeated clearly.

LINKS WITH HOME
If the child that you are targeting is more vocal at home than in the setting, lend the family a tape recorder or blank tape. Ask them to record their child speaking or singing at home so that you can hear their level of language and build on it in your setting.

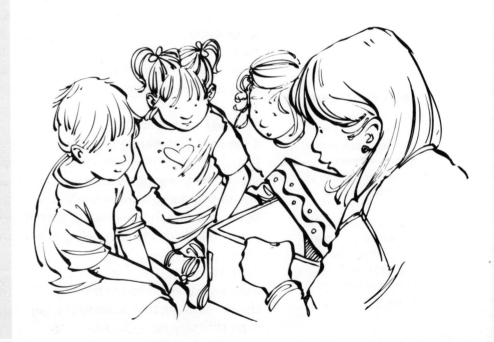

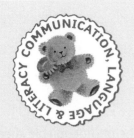

Past and present

Group size
Four to six children.

What you need
A whiteboard; marker pen; cards; thick felt-tipped pen; Blu-Tack.

What to do
Carry out this activity on a Tuesday, Wednesday or Thursday as part of a key worker session, or if any of the children are starting and finishing their sessions in 'home base' groups where they meet with their special teacher or adult.

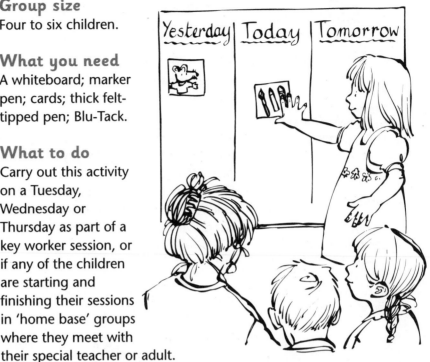

Sit in a circle with the children and start by talking about what the children did yesterday. Which activity did they enjoy the most? Take out the cards and draw little pictures to represent what the children tell you, for example, a child painting, a model, a story character.

Talk about the activities that you have planned for the children today. What would the group like to do today? Again, draw pictures on cards to represent each child's ideas and plans.

Finally, introduce new activities that you are planning for tomorrow and do the same. Keep track of the children's ideas as they talk by placing the cards representing their own ideas in front of them.

Now divide your whiteboard into three sections – 'Yesterday', 'Today' and 'Tomorrow'. Go around the circle, inviting each child to put up the activity that they enjoyed about yesterday on the whiteboard with Blu-Tack. Repeat for 'Today', then 'Tomorrow'. Revise the concepts by asking the children, 'What did you do yesterday?', 'What will you do tomorrow?' and so on.

Special support
Some children with language difficulties find it hard to understand the sequences of time. Use the planning board to give the child that you are targeting a visual sequence of what is going to happen during each session. Use pictures, from left to right, illustrating circle time, sand and water play, painting, outdoor play, snack time and so on. Always make sure that the child knows what to do and what to do next. Encourage 'doing and reviewing'.

Extension
Let the children draw their own pictures. Extend questioning to include 'When?' questions, for example, 'When are you going to paint?'.

LEARNING OBJECTIVE FOR ALL THE CHILDREN
● to show an understanding of the sequence of events.

INDIVIDUAL LEARNING TARGET
● to talk about events which happen 'yesterday', 'today' and 'tomorrow'.

LINKS WITH HOME
Suggest to parents and carers that they use visual timetables for routines at home.

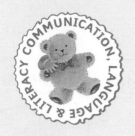

LEARNING OBJECTIVE FOR ALL THE CHILDREN
● to use a pencil and hold it effectively to form recognizable letters.

INDIVIDUAL LEARNING TARGETS
● to hold a pencil correctly
● to repeat a letter sound.

LINKS WITH HOME
Ask the parents or carers of the child that you are targeting to help them write their name by writing it in yellow felt-tipped pen and then inviting the child to copy over it.

Give me a B!

Group size
Two or three children.

What you need
Sheets of paper; washable felt-tipped pens; the photocopiable sheet on page 88.

What to do
Introduce this activity once you have become familiar with the 'Buzzy bee' activity on page 35. Sit with the children around a table and sing 'The buzzy bee song' on the photocopiable sheet together. Show the children how to write the letter for each verse, starting with 'z'. Use hand over hand to model the straight or circular movement. Once the children are beginning to make the movement independently, draw a 'z' or 'b' in yellow felt-tipped pen and invite them to copy over the top. Finally, encourage each child to copy the letter independently, covering their page with different-coloured letters.

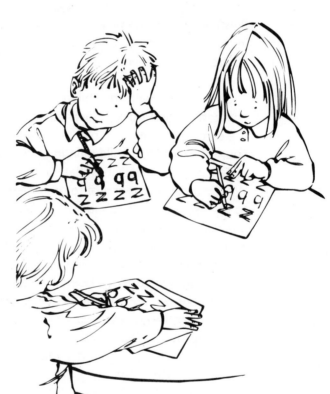

Special support
Encourage the child that you are targeting to practise saying the sound as they write the letter. Keep the activity fun and motivating. If the child has difficulty in holding a pen or pencil correctly, use a triangular pen or grip to encourage the correct 'tripod' hold (see page 96).

Extension
Challenge the children to practise the letters that they have written by chanting 'Give me a "i"' (saying the letter sound, not its name), 'Give me a "s"' and so on.

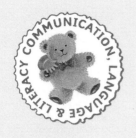

LEARNING OBJECTIVE FOR ALL THE CHILDREN
● to experiment with sounds and signs.

INDIVIDUAL LEARNING TARGET
● to sign clearly and visibly.

LINKS WITH HOME
Ask the parents or carers of the targeted child which signs they are learning and practising. Draw up a sheet of these and share it with your colleagues in the setting.

Dog: beg with two 'paws' up (indexes and middle fingers).
Cat: preen your whiskers (indexes and middle fingers).
Pig: a fist on your nose with a screwing movement.
Sheep: little fingers at the sides of your face moving outwards to draw a curly fleece.
Cow: two fists on your brow, moving up in the shape of two horns.
Horse: two fingers astride one finger and trotting twice only.

Old MacDonald's Makaton farm

Group size
Eight to ten children.

What you need
Pictures and toys or models of farm animals.

What to do
If you have a child who is learning to use Makaton sign language, perhaps because of their speech and language difficulty or hearing impairment, use this activity as a 'warm-up' song during music or circle time. You will find a useful contact address on page 96. Talk to parents, carers or the visiting speech and language therapist about the signs the child is using and ask them to demonstrate them to you.

Sing 'Old MacDonald Had a Farm'. Stop at the point where you need to think of an animal and invite the children to give you some suggestions. Ask, 'What does a cow say?', 'Can you remember the sign for cow?' and so on. Have just one animal for each verse so as not to burden the children's memories at this stage.

Special support
Spend an individual session teaching the Makaton signs to the child that you are targeting and for whom these have been recommended. Sit opposite the child, share a picture or small toy model of each animal and exaggerate the sign with your hands. Then help the child to make the sign by guiding hand over hand if necessary. Say the animal's name as you teach the sign. Start by introducing one sign for a favourite animal and then build up the repertoire gradually.

Extension
Encourage the children to invent new versions of 'Old MacDonald Had a Farm', for example, 'Old MacDonald had a jungle'. Invite them to give you suggestions for actions and sounds to go with the verses.

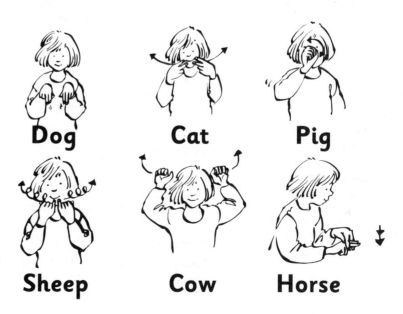

Dog   Cat   Pig

Sheep   Cow   Horse

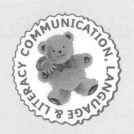

LEARNING OBJECTIVE FOR ALL THE CHILDREN
● to hear and say the middle and final sounds in words.

INDIVIDUAL LEARNING TARGET
● to develop an awareness of words which sound the same.

Rhyme time

Group size
Up to 20 children.

What you need
Just the children.

What to do
Sit with the children in a circle. Sing a well-known action song that has rhyming words such as 'This Old Man'.

> This old man, he played one,
> He played nick-nack on my...
> With a nick-nack, paddy-whack,
> Give the dog a bone,
> This old man came rolling home! (and so on)
> (Traditional)

When you reach the rhyming word, pause, look puzzled and ask the children for suggestions. Explain that you want a word that sounds like 'one' or 'two'. The children will offer many words that do not rhyme, for example 'tree' to rhyme with 'two'. In this case, say the pairs together and ask the children if the words sound the same, for example, 'two... tree... two... tree'. Build up the song verse by verse until you have found rhyming words for each one.

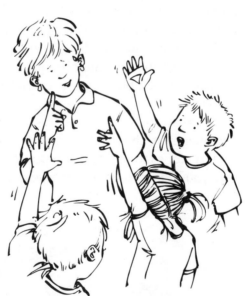

Special support
Children with speech and language difficulties may find rhyming activities particularly hard to accomplish. Research has linked this difficulty in 'phonological awareness' to specific literacy or 'dyslexic' difficulties later on. Use your mouth movements to really emphasize the sounds to the children to make the activity easier. Spend time with the child that you are targeting enjoying rhymes and picture poetry in the book corner.

Extension
Give the children two words such as 'shoe' and 'shell', or 'shoe' and 'two'. Ask the group whether these words sound the same or if they rhyme. For children who are very 'phonically aware', build up to three words, such as 'shoe', 'goat' and 'two' and ask them which two sound the same.

LINKS WITH HOME
Write out familiar nursery rhymes for parents and carers to enjoy with their children at home.

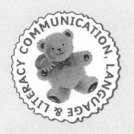

Lucky labels

Group size
Whole group.

What you need
Self-adhesive name labels; name cards; washable felt-tipped pens; small stickers.

What to do
Before you start this activity, write each child's first name clearly on a sticker and then on a piece of card.

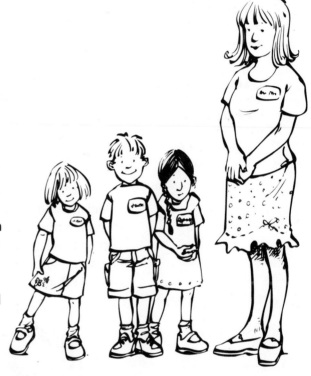

Carry out this activity on a day when you have a visitor in the setting, or at a time when many of the children are still new. Tell the children that you would like each of them to wear a label with their name on so that the visitor will know what to call them.

Invite two or three children at a time to come to find their name labels. Show them the sticky labels and see if they identify theirs, helping them if you need to.

The next day, ask the children to find their name labels again.

After a few days, provide the children with blank sticky labels. Invite each child to find their name from your selection of name cards and to copy it onto their label. Provide small stickers for the children to decorate and personalize their labels.

Special support
If necessary, provide hand-over-hand support when the children copy their names, or write their names in yellow felt-tipped pen for them to copy over. Use larger labels if you need to. If the child that you are targeting has difficulty in finding their name label, reduce the choice by providing just two or three very different names to choose from. Encourage the child to say their name as they read it. Echo it back clearly for them to listen to.

Extension
Let the children write their names independently and clearly. Can they find other children's names, too? How many names can they read now?

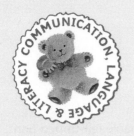

You spy, too

Group size
Six children.

What you need
Six familiar objects with clear consonant word beginnings such as a cup, brick, train, lollipop, toy dog and glove; six cards, approximately A5 format; pens.

What to do
Write the initial letter of each object on one side of each card, for example, 'c', 'b', 't', 'l', 'd' and 'g'. On the other side of each card, draw a picture of the corresponding object.

Sit with the children in a circle on the floor. Place the six objects and the six cards, letter side up, on the floor in the centre. Invite the child that you are targeting to sit beside you and be your helper.

Ask the child to choose one of the objects and to whisper it to you. Talk quietly to the child and ask what sound the object begins with, prompting if you need to. Once you have decided together what the initial sound is, tell all the children that (child's name) has chosen something that begins with (first letter of the object). Ask the targeted child to tell all the children the initial sound. Invite the rest of the group to guess what the object is and also to identify the written letter that makes that sound. Repeat for all the objects and sounds.

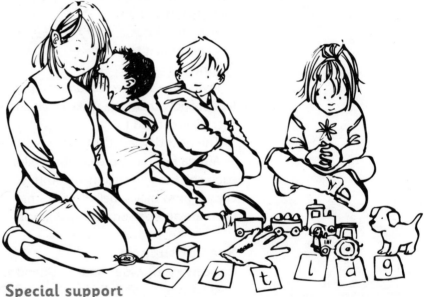

Special support
Once the child that you are targeting has become used to the pictures, cards and sounds, dispense with the objects and use the cards to help the child remember their letter sounds. Show the child a card with the letter side facing them. If they cannot remember what it says, let them turn the card over and remember the initial sound of the object.

Extension
Write whole words for the objects chosen instead of just initial sounds on one side of the card.

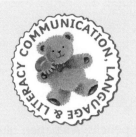

LEARNING OBJECTIVE FOR ALL THE CHILDREN
● to retell narratives in the correct sequence, drawing on the language patterns of words.

INDIVIDUAL LEARNING TARGET
● to place story pictures in the correct sequence.

Story chains

Group size
Three or four children.

What you need
The photocopiable sheet on page 89; cards; pens; scissors (adult use).

What to do
Copy the photocopiable sheet onto card and cut out the four pictures. Sit around a table with the children and show them the pictures one at a time, but not in the correct order. Ask the group what is happening in each picture. Once you have talked about a picture, place it on the table so that the children can still see it. When all four pictures are laid out, invite the child that you are targeting to arrange the cards in the correct story sequence, from left to right across the table, with everyone helping. Now invite the child to retell you the story as it happened, pointing to each picture in turn.

Make your own story chains and talk about them together as you arrange them.

Special support
Sometimes children with language difficulties find it hard to understand sequences. Help the child that you are targeting to talk about who was involved, where they are, what they are doing and what might happen next. Be aware that they might struggle with the 'who/where/what' words themselves. If so, be ready to help them put their thoughts into words and to remember them long enough to sequence the pictures.

Extension
Let the children make up their own picture sequences and help them to show them to one another.

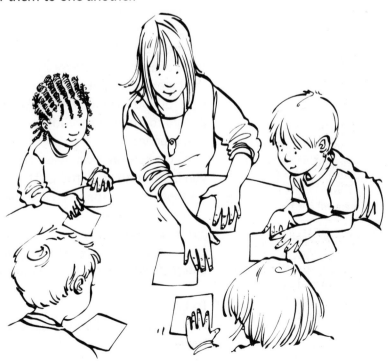

LINKS WITH HOME
Let the child that you are targeting take home a pack of simple sequences and ask their parents or carers to practise them with their child.

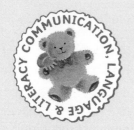

Good report

Group size
Whole group.

What you need
A tape recorder; blank tape; A4 paper; pens; pencils; A3 paper; glue; newspaper.

What to do
Gather the children together in a circle and show them your newspaper. Pass it around the group and ask questions such as, 'What is a newspaper for?', 'What does it tell you?', 'If we wanted to tell people all about us and our setting, what things could we put in our own newspaper?' and so on.

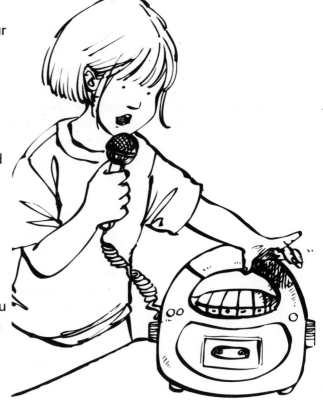

Then suggest to the children that you are going to make a newspaper for parents and carers and collect ideas from the group. Encourage the children to help you think of a suitable title for the newspaper. Show the group how to use the tape recorder and encourage each child to say something on the tape for you to write in the newspaper. Then invite them to draw a picture to go with their idea. Support them as they put their thoughts into practice.

As the session progresses, encourage each child to stay beside you as you listen to their words on the tape and you write them onto a large A3 sheet of 'newspaper'. Glue their picture underneath their words.

Special support
Help the child that you are targeting to put their thoughts into a short complete sentence. Play the tape back and praise their attempts.

Extension
Encourage the children to each try to write their own simple report for the newspaper.

LEARNING OBJECTIVES FOR ALL THE CHILDREN
- to use talk to organise, sequence and clarify events
- to attempt writing to report an event.

INDIVIDUAL LEARNING TARGET
- to put together a short sentence.

LINKS WITH HOME
Copy the newspaper onto A3 paper for each child and let them take it home. Ask parents and carers to read through the newspaper with their children and to encourage them to talk about it.

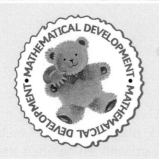

MATHEMATICAL DEVELOPMENT

This chapter encourages all the children's mathematical development. There are ideas for making learning opportunities as 'concrete' as possible, particularly for those children who find abstract language hard to understand.

Over and under the bridge

Group size
Up to six children.

What you need
The Three Billy Goats Gruff (Traditional); a simple plank bridge made from three pieces of thick wood; three toy goats; something monster-like to represent the troll.

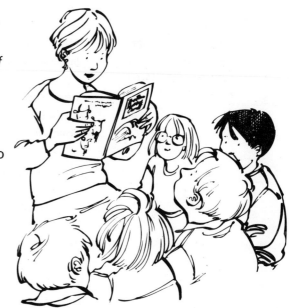

What to do
Read the story of *The Three Billy Goats Gruff* to the children and look at the pictures together. Encourage the group to help you re-enact the story with the props. Ask one child to construct the bridge, another to place the troll under the bridge and the other children to make a goat 'trip-trap-trip-trap' over the bridge.

Invite the child that you are targeting to place the troll over the bridge as it creeps out to catch one of the goats, and then to hide the goat under the bridge once it has been caught. Look for opportunities to reinforce the words 'under' and 'over' as your story progresses.

Special support
Before you carry out the activity, set up a short individual session with the child that you are targeting using a bridge, goat and troll to familiarize the child with the words 'over' and 'under'. After the activity, set up a short individual session with a toy chair and small toy to assess whether the child can extend their learning to a new situation – for example, can they put the cat 'under' the chair?.

Extension
Provide building blocks and toy animals for the children to play imaginatively and act out their own versions of the story with. Make your own 'lift-the-flap' book so that the children can lift the flap to see what is under the bridge.

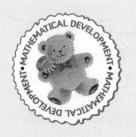

LEARNING OBJECTIVE FOR ALL THE CHILDREN
● to say and use number names in order.

INDIVIDUAL LEARNING TARGET
● to place numbers 1 to 3 in their correct order.

Number line

Group size
Whole group.

What you need
A set of coloured magnetic numbers, 1 to 5; magnetic board or metallic surface such as a fridge door; thin strip of card with ten numbers the same size and colour as the magnetic shapes; thin strip of card with the outlines of the numbers on.

What to do
Tell the children that you have muddled up all the magnetic numbers on the board. Can anyone sort them out? Invite the children to come and tell you when the numbers are in the correct order, and give successful children a sticker or celebratory stamp. This will help you to notice which children can already order their numbers and those who need support. The task should also inspire discussion as the children work together to solve the problem. If some children find this difficult, start with fewer numbers, for example, 1 to 3.

Special support
For those children who are still learning to order numbers, show them how to place the strip of coloured numbers on the board and match

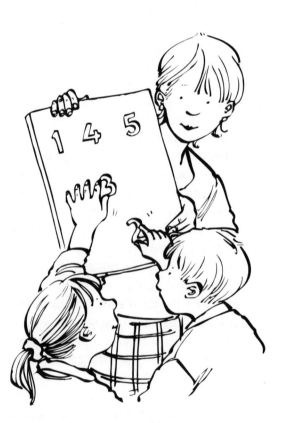

the numbers onto it. Again, you can start with fewer numbers and a shorter strip (such as 1 to 3) until the task becomes easy. Once the children are able to do this, challenge them to use the strip with the outline of the numbers (which are not coloured). As a further step, hold the strip beside the numbers so that the children copy underneath rather than match one-to-one.

Extension
Jumble up the numbers 1 to 9 and challenge the children to rearrange them in the correct order. Give a short sequence, for example, 4, 5, (blank), 7 and encourage them to add the missing number.

LINKS WITH HOME
Encourage parents and carers to buy a set of magnetic numbers for their fridge door and suggest simple number activities for them to try with their children.

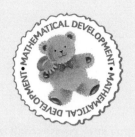

LEARNING OBJECTIVE FOR ALL THE CHILDREN
● to use everyday words to describe position, including ordinal numbers.

INDIVIDUAL LEARNING TARGET
● to use the words 'first' and 'last'.

Tailback

Group size
Six children.

What you need
An assortment of six toy vehicles; floor space; large sheet of paper; thick felt-tipped pen.

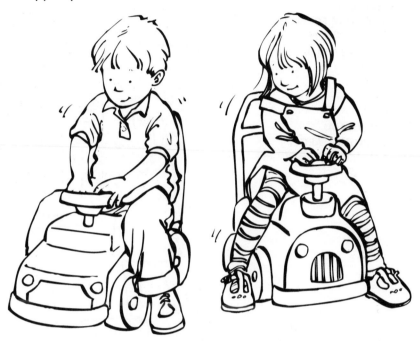

What to do
Gather the children in a circle and spread the large sheet of paper on the floor. Tell the children a story about each vehicle, drawing a shed, a garage or a yard for each vehicle to park in around the edge of the paper. Draw a road just wide enough to take the vehicles, leading from each house to a petrol station in the middle of town. Make all six roads converge into one before they come up to the garage. Draw roads leading back to the six homes from the other side of the petrol station.

Give each child a toy vehicle and invite one child to 'drive' their vehicle all the way to the petrol station and park at the entrance. Continue your narration as each child in turn 'drives' their vehicle into town, joining the queue for the petrol station! You will now have six vehicles in a row. Challenge the children in turn to show you the first/last/second/fourth/third/fifth vehicle in the queue. As each vehicle in turn 'fills up with petrol' and drives home, ask, 'Who is first/last/second/fourth/third/fifth now?'.

Special support
Start by giving the child that you are targeting an easy concept such as 'first' and then build up to other position words.

Extension
Invite the children to say the ordinal numbers (first, second, third and so on) up to tenth.

LINKS WITH HOME
Give each child a copy of the photocopiable sheet on page 90 to take home. Invite parents and carers to read it to their children and to help them complete it.

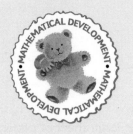

Number socks

Group size
Two or three children.

What you need
Three colourful adult-sized socks; a low washing line; pegs; small round pebbles.

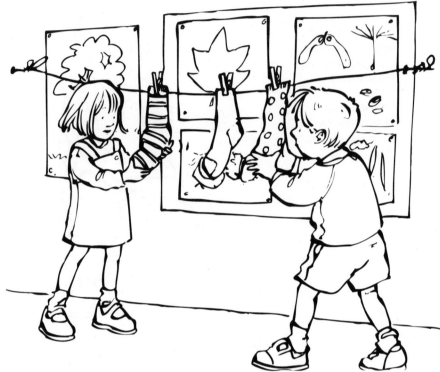

What to do
Hang the washing line up at one end of your room at the children's height but just in front of a wall so that they do not bump into it. Peg the three socks in a row. Ask the children to place one pebble in the first sock, two pebbles in the second sock and three pebbles in the third sock. Invite them to cover their eyes while you rearrange the socks. Ask, 'Can you feel how many pebbles there are in each sock?', 'How many pebbles would there be if you added one more?' and 'How many pebbles would there be if you took one away?'. Work it out together by counting.

Special support
Start by giving the child that you are targeting the sock with one pebble in. Then give them a sock with one pebble in and a sock with three pebbles in. Encourage them to identify which sock has 'more' in and which sock has 'less' in. Some children with language and communication difficulties are very good at counting by rote but may find the more abstract concepts of 'more' and 'less' more difficult.

Extension
When the children can identify 'more' and 'less', build up the number of socks and pebbles to five. Hang the socks up in any order and challenge the children to peg them in the correct order.

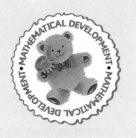

LEARNING OBJECTIVE FOR ALL THE CHILDREN
● to recognize and re-create simple patterns.

INDIVIDUAL LEARNING TARGET
● to identify and name 'high' and 'low'.

Highs and lows

Group size
Two or three children.

What you need
Building blocks; solid floor or low surface to build on; chalk.

What to do
Tell the children that you are going to build a street of buildings. Talk together as you draw a chalk line to represent the long street where the buildings are going to go. Show the children how they can make 'high' houses and 'low' houses by stacking the bricks. Build one high and one low next to each other. Invite the children to continue the pattern and to build a row of houses that are high, then low, then high, then low, all along the street.

Special support
Before you carry out the activity, have a short individual session with the child that you are targeting. Build two towers and ask, 'Which one is the high tower?' and 'Which one is the low tower?'. Help the child by pointing if you need to. Keep it fun and praise warmly. Now move some bricks from the high tower to the low tower, making that one into the new high tower. Ask, 'Which is the high tower now?' and so on.

Extension
Introduce new patterns for the children to follow, for example, a red house, a blue house, a yellow house, a red house, and so on. Let the children paint the street of houses on a long wall frieze.

LINKS WITH HOME
Ask parents and carers to find opportunities to talk about 'high' and 'low' with their children and to point out high and low buildings on their journey to and from your setting.

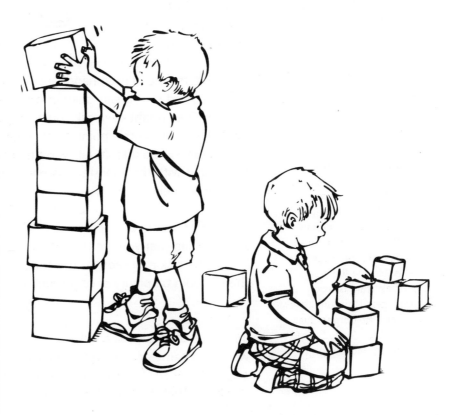

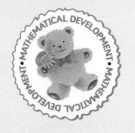

Shopping basket

Group size
Three or four children.

What you need
Two identical baskets; selection of tinned food, packages, toys and other assorted items for a shopping bag; set of bathroom scales.

What to do
Before starting the activity, fill up both baskets with your selection of items, so that one basket is a lot heavier than the other. Invite the children to lift the baskets and tell you which is the heavier one and which is the lighter one. Then challenge the children to make the two baskets weigh the same and support them as

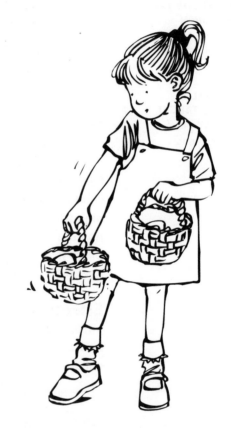

they work out different ways to do this. The children might hold the two baskets, one in each hand, and compare them, or they may empty them out and start again, sharing out the heavy cans and the light objects. They might even ask you if you have any scales. Inject your own ideas at a suitable point where it would extend their own thinking. Encourage the children to talk and discuss as they work out the problem. Help them with the final stages if necessary so that they complete the task successfully.

Special support
Ask the child that you are targeting to tell you which basket is the heavy one as the task proceeds. As the children experiment with the items, there should be plenty of opportunities to reinforce this concept.

Extension
Introduce the scales as another method of finding out whether things weigh the same or not. Set up another activity with balance scales and containers to see whether the children can fill the containers with small objects so that they weigh the same.

LEARNING OBJECTIVES FOR ALL THE CHILDREN
● to use the language 'heavier' or 'lighter' in practical activities and discussion
● to begin to use the vocabulary involved in addition and subtraction.

INDIVIDUAL LEARNING TARGET
● to identify and name 'heavy'.

LINKS WITH HOME
Ask parents and carers to encourage their children to find three objects around the house which are 'heavy' and three which are 'light'. If their child is being targeted for language help, encourage them to teach 'heavy' first, before moving on to 'light'.

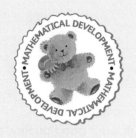

LEARNING OBJECTIVE FOR ALL THE CHILDREN

● to use language such as 'circle' and 'round'.

INDIVIDUAL LEARNING TARGET

● to identify and name a 'circle' shape.

All around

Group size
Four to six children.

What you need
Large paper plates; sticky paper shapes; paints; felt-tipped pens; pencils; cotton; sticky tape.

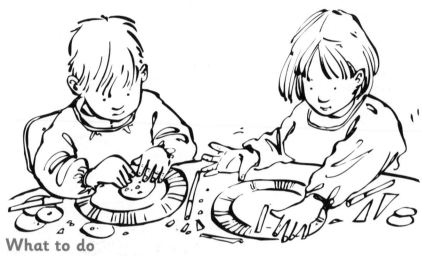

What to do
Gather the children together and show them one of the paper plates. Talk together about what shape it is. Use the words 'round' and 'circle'. Now invite the children to look around the room from where they are sitting. Can they see anything else that is round? They might be able to see a clock-face, plate of biscuits, ball, hoop, the end of a paper roll, a doorknob or a wheel. Now send the group out around the room, inviting each child to come back and tell you about something round which they saw. Then gather a few round objects together so that you can talk about them.

Provide sticky paper shapes, paints and felt-tipped pens and let the children draw pictures on paper plates to represent the round things that they have seen. They might draw a clock-face or stick paper shapes on to represent the plate of biscuits. Attach a piece of cotton to each 'round' picture and suspend them from the ceiling to make a round mobile which twists and turns.

Special support
Encourage the child that you are targeting to hold their plate near to an object as you trace the shape of the object with your finger. Ask them, 'Is it round? They will find the direct comparison easier. Continue to use the words 'round' and 'circle' where new opportunities arise over the next few days until the child has linked the abstract words to the circular images.

Extension
Introduce solid three-dimensional shapes such as cylinders, cones, pyramids and cuboids. Encourage the children to manipulate them and count any 'round' sides.

LINKS WITH HOME
Ask parents and carers to let their children bring one round object into the setting the next day.

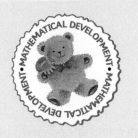

LEARNING OBJECTIVE FOR ALL THE CHILDREN
● to recognize numerals 1 to 9.

INDIVIDUAL LEARNING TARGET
● to name '1', '2' and '3'.

LINKS WITH HOME
Let the children take turns at bringing the book home, or invite parents and carers to look through it with their children at home time. Tell them which sections of the book you would like them to share with their children and invite them to encourage their children to touch objects in the larger sets as they count out loud.

Number splits

Group size
Two children.

What you need
A large, spiral-bound notebook; scissors (adult use); good quality, plain art paper; brightly coloured washable felt-tipped pens; glue.

What to do
Before you begin, leave one complete page at the front and the back of the notebook and then cut across the centre of all the other pages, separating the top halves of the pages from the bottom halves. The children will enjoy sitting beside you as you make this split book.

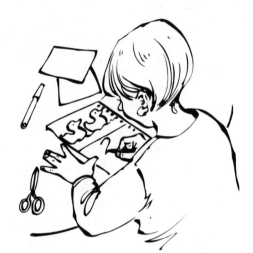

Invite the child that you are targeting and a friend to sit beside you and to help. Turn to the first split page. Write a large number '1' on the bottom half of the page. Ask the children to give you ideas of what you can draw on the top half, for example, one cat.

On the next page, write the number '2' on the bottom half and again ask for ideas for two objects to draw on the top half. Encourage the children to help by counting and colouring. On the next page, write the number '3' and then have another ten pages or so with '1', '2' or '3' on. Move on to pages '4' and '5' and gradually build your book up to sets of '9' and '10'. Invite different children to come and help as the book makes progress over a number of sessions.

If you do not feel comfortable drawing, cut and stick pictures instead, or use self-adhesive stickers.

When the book is complete, encourage the children to match the correct number to the corresponding set of objects by turning and matching split pages.

Special support
Repeating the numbers on different pages allows for the repetition that many children with learning and language difficulties need.

Concentrate on the early pages with numbers up to '3' for the child that you are targeting until these are known and then move on to the rest of the book.

Extension
Encourage the children to make up their own pages in the book.

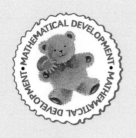

Ticket queue

Group size
Whole group.

What you need
A low table and chair; pieces of paper; scissors; pencils; toy cash register or bus conductor's ticket machine; bus stop sign; low chairs; hats for the bus driver and conductor; other props such as baskets, dressing-up clothes, toy cameras and so on.

What to do
Gather the children together and talk about travelling on a bus. Encourage them to talk about what happens and help them to sequence their ideas. First, they have to queue up at the bus stop, then they have to hold their hands out for the bus to stop, then they get on and buy a ticket.

Suggest that you create a 'bus' for your setting. Show the children how they can set up a ticket office, how to make bus tickets and how to arrange the chairs in a row to make the bus. Stay in their game as they organize themselves into passengers, conductor and driver. Encourage the use of the dressing-up clothes and other items. As you queue or take your seat, look for opportunities to ask, 'Who is sitting behind me?', 'Who is in front of me?' and so on. Leave the children to develop the game independently.

Special support
Reinforce the words 'behind' and 'in front of' naturally as the game progresses.

Extension
Introduce money and priced tickets for the children to practise counting 1p and 2p coins.

LEARNING OBJECTIVE FOR ALL THE CHILDREN
● to use everyday words to describe position.

INDIVIDUAL LEARNING TARGET
● to identify and respond to 'in front of' and 'behind'.

LINKS WITH HOME
Ask the parents or carers of the child that you are targeting to play a simple game with a soft toy and a cardboard box. Encourage them to ask their child to hide Teddy 'behind' or 'in front of' the box, helping if they have to and warmly praising the child's success.

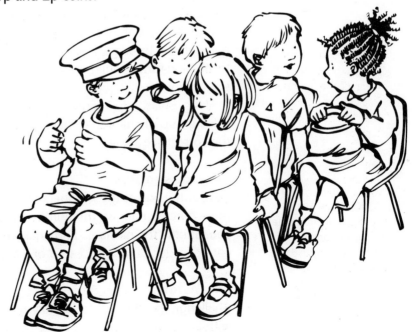

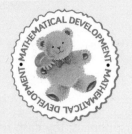

LEARNING OBJECTIVES FOR ALL THE CHILDREN
● to recognize and order numerals 1 to 9
● to count reliably from 1 to 9.

INDIVIDUAL LEARNING TARGETS
● to remember the sequence 1 to 9 when counting
● to say the number names clearly.

Number dangles

Group size
Ten children.

What you need
Sheets of stiff card; fine and rough sandpaper; metallic and reflective paper and card; glue; spreaders; sparkly stickers; sequins; dried red and green lentils; scissors (adult use); washing line; pegs.

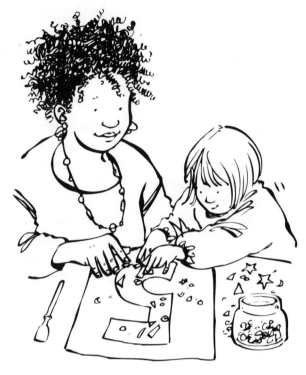

What to do
Draw the outline of the numerals 1 to 9, approximately 30cm high, onto card. Invite one or two children at a time to join you at a table. Encourage them to help you make a numeral by sticking materials within the outline of the numeral. Ask them to choose reflective paper and sparkly decorations to stick onto the numeral to make it as glittery and attractive as possible. Leave the decorated numbers to dry.

Once the glue has dried, cut the shape of the number out. Invite the child or children to come back to the table and decorate the reverse side of the numeral by painting it with glue and sprinkling on green or red lentils. Alternatively, help them to cut around a sandpaper number and to glue iy onto the reverse side of the numeral. Each decorated numeral will then have one shiny and reflective side, and one dull but tactile side for the children to feel. Again, place the numbers on one side to dry.

Hang a washing line up at the children's height, just in front of a wall. Ask a group of children to help you identify and peg up the numbers in the correct sequence.

Special support
Look at the line of the numbers with the child you are targeting and let them practise naming the numbers independently, or repeating after you. Shuffle the numbers and challenge the child to put them in the correct order. Start with 1 to 3 or 1 to 5 if necessary.

Extension
Challenge the children to identify the number shapes by touching them with their eyes closed.

LINKS WITH HOME
Send a numeral home and invite parents and carers to help their children to find a set of this number of similar objects.

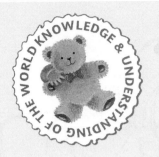

KNOWLEDGE AND UNDERSTANDING OF THE WORLD

This chapter will help all the children to develop knowledge and understanding of their world, with ideas to encourage less able children to ask and respond to questions appropriately.

Musical know-how

Group size
Up to 24 children.

What you need
A musician to demonstrate and explain an instrument, for example, someone who plays the African drums, a member of a steel band, a folk musician, a saxophonist, or a French-horn player.

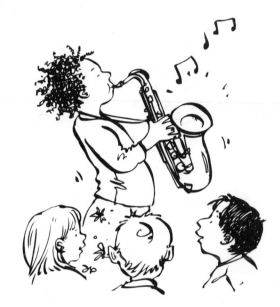

What to do
Suggest to the musician that they show the children their instrument first. Then invite discussion from the children as to what noise it might make and how to make sounds with it. Explain to the children that the musician is going to play their instrument for them. Be aware that some children find loud noises alarming and might prefer to watch or listen from a neighbouring room. Encourage the children to listen to the sound of the instrument and invite them to ask their own questions of the musician.

Encourage the children to think about how the sounds are made. Should this instrument be beaten like a drum, shaken like a shaker or blown like a whistle? Encourage the children to think of helpful questions to ask and support them as they address the musician. Keep the session fairly brief and end while the children are still interested.

Special support
Help the child that you are targeting to ask one of the first questions such as 'What is it?'. Follow up with helping them to use this question to find out the names of some simple percussion instruments in your music box.

Extension
Carry out a project on musical sounds and instruments. Make up a music table and enjoy a 'jam session' with a musical tape and plenty of percussion instruments.

LEARNING OBJECTIVE FOR ALL THE CHILDREN
● to ask questions about why things happen and how things work.

INDIVIDUAL LEARNING TARGET
● to ask 'What...?' questions.

LINKS WITH HOME
Ask the parents or carers of the child that you are targeting to play a simple game with them. They should place four familiar items onto a table and ask the child in turn, 'What is this?'. Then they should encourage their child to ask them instead, using the 'What...?' question.

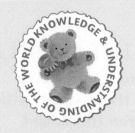

Why not?

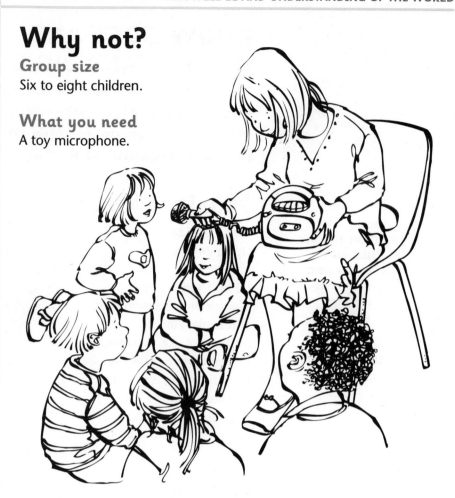

Group size
Six to eight children.

What you need
A toy microphone.

What to do
Gather the children in a circle. Pretend that you are making a news programme for television. Ask, 'Has anyone seen the news on television?', 'Have you seen how people talk to each other and answer questions?', 'Do you think this a good way to find things out?' and so on. Go around the circle and encourage each child to think of a question.

Now pretend to be an interviewer. Hold up your microphone to each child in turn as you ask a simple question, for example, 'What is your name?' or 'How old are you?'. Invite the children to take turns at being an interviewer and support them as they move around the circle and ask each child a question. Provide some ideas if they are unsure. Encourage the 'interviewer' to repeat back the answer and use your commentary to make it feel like a television recording, for example, 'So *this* is Bethany Thomson and she is four years old', 'This is interesting! Sultan has come to the settting today to make a *big red train*' and so on.

Special support
If the child that you are targeting has difficulty in understanding question words such as 'why' and 'when', use this activity to focus on a certain word. Support them as they ask each of the other children, 'Why do you come to nursery?', encouraging them to listen to the reply and tell you the answer.

Extension
Provide a tape recorder for the children to interview one another.

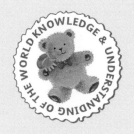

LEARNING OBJECTIVE FOR ALL THE CHILDREN
● to find out about past and present events in their own lives.

INDIVIDUAL LEARNING TARGET
● to talk about their personal experiences in a small group.

This is me

Group size
Three or four children.

What you need
Two or three photographs of each child showing them at different stages of their lives brought in from home; photograph album with self-adhesive pages; small pieces of paper; pen.

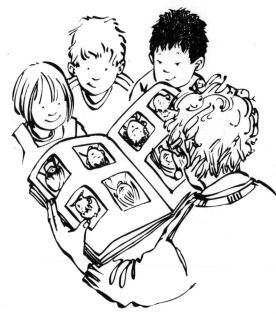

What to do
Tell parents and carers that you are going to carry out a project on 'All about me' and ask them to help their children to choose two or three photographs showing themselves as babies and toddlers, or on particular occasions or holidays. Ask them to write their children's names on the back of the photographs and a few words about the situation. Assure them that you will return the photographs afterwards. Not every child will be able to bring in photographs so make sure that you have some of your own that you have taken of the children over the past few months.

Sit down with individual children to share their photographs and mount them in your album so that each child has a section of a page. Ask them what they would like you to write on a small piece of paper as a caption for each photograph.

When you have photographs from three or four children, sit down as a group and share them together. Encourage the children to talk about the past, present and future. If they find tenses difficult such as 'I used to live', 'I lived', 'I live' and 'I will live', then gently repeat back to them correctly what they are trying to say.

Continue with your album until you have a section for everybody. Use the photographs that you have taken in the setting for those children who did not bring any of their own.

Special support
Use the album as a talking point to encourage the child that you are targeting to talk about their past experiences. Again, gently echo back to the child what they are trying to say to you if it is not clear or if it is grammatically incorrect.

Extension
Encourage the children to imagine and draw themselves as six-year-olds, as eleven-year-olds or even as grown-ups! Talk about what they have drawn.

LINKS WITH HOME
Thank parents and carers for supplying the photographs and encourage them to look through the album in your setting and talk about it with their children.

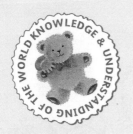

LEARNING OBJECTIVE FOR ALL THE CHILDREN
● to find out about and identify some of the features of living things.

INDIVIDUAL LEARNING TARGETS
● to point to and name body parts
● to improve eye contact.

LINKS WITH HOME
Ask parents and carers to practise learning body parts with their children by challenging them to 'show me your *nose*' and so on and to make a game of it.

Body beautiful

Group size
Even numbers of children up to 12.

What to do
Familiarize yourself with the rhyme below.

Nose, nose, show me your nose!
The colder it gets, the more it blows!
Toe, toe, show me your toe!
Then wiggle and jiggle it down below!
Ear, ear, show me an ear!
They hold on your specs and they help you to hear!
Eye, eye, show me an eye!
They help you to watch everybody go by!
Chin, chin, show me your chin!
You lower it downwards to let your food in!
Tummy, tummy, show me your tummy!
We give it a tickle and make it feel funny!

Hannah Mortimer

Encourage the children to sit on the floor, each facing a partner. Introduce the rhyme and encourage the children to point to their own body parts at the appropriate times. Emphasize the key words (the body parts) as you sing. Then repeat the rhyme, encouraging the children to point gently to the body parts of their partners in each verse.

Special support
This rhyme emphasizes the body parts clearly for those children with speech and language difficulties. Practise the pointing actions with a mirror and a large teddy bear and encourage eye contact as you partner the child that you are targeting. The child should then be ready to join in with a partner.

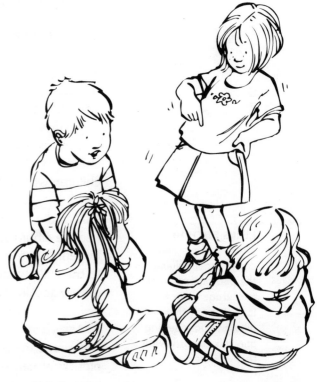

Extension
Ask the children to suggest ideas for more verses.

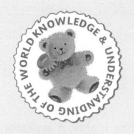

Gone fishing

Group size
Two or three children.

What you need
The photocopiable sheet on page 91; scissors; washable felt-tipped pens; metallic paper clips; length of thin dowel approximately 30cm long; string; small magnet; large sheet of blue paper; low table.

What to do
Make two A3 copies of the photocopiable sheet. Sit down with some of the more able children and colour in the fish in bright colours. You will need two identical sets of coloured fish so that the fish on one sheet corresponds exactly with the fish on the other sheet. Talk about 'same' and 'different' as you work together.

Carefully cut out the fish and attach a paper clip to the mouth of each one. Make a 'fishing line' by tying string to the magnet and dangling it from one end of the piece of dowelling. Arrange all the fish on a sheet of blue paper placed on a low table to represent 'the sea'.

Gather two or three children together and show them how they can use the rod to 'catch' the fish. As each child catches a fish, encourage them to catch another just the same. Let the children take turns until all the fish are caught.

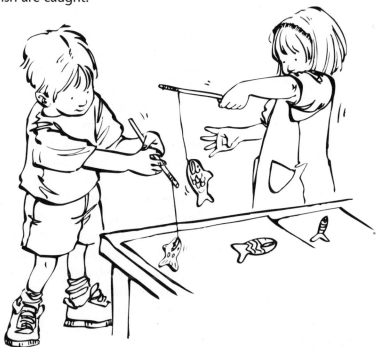

Special support
Emphasize the key words 'same' and 'different' as you talk and ask the child that you are targeting to judge whether the two fish caught by any of his friends are the same. If so, the child can act as your helper and say 'Well done!'.

Extension
Let the children make up their own fish patterns for the fishing game.

LEARNING OBJECTIVE FOR ALL THE CHILDREN
● to look closely at similarities and differences.

INDIVIDUAL LEARNING TARGET
● to respond appropriately to the words 'same' and 'different'.

LINKS WITH HOME
Use the fishing game for parents and carers to teach things at home. They can be used to help their children match pictures, letters, sets of objects and words. Make up sets of 'fish' for the children to take home and suggest ideas to parents and carers for using them.

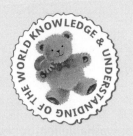

LEARNING OBJECTIVES FOR ALL THE CHILDREN
● to investigate natural materials
● to look closely at change.

INDIVIDUAL LEARNING TARGET
● to use the words 'wet', 'dry', 'cold' and 'hot'.

LINKS WITH HOME
Ask parents and carers to talk with their children about their fridge at home and ask questions such as, 'What foods need to be kept in there?', 'Where is the ice made?', 'Why does the door need to stay shut?' and so on.

Ice cubes

Group size
Four to six children.

What you need
Food colouring; ice-cube trays; novelty ice-cube maker, if available; drinking water; clear plastic tumblers and bowls; natural fruit juices; pieces of fruit; tray for each child; low table.

What to do
Make up some trays of ice cubes in advance. One tray should be colourless drinking water and the others can be drinking water coloured with different food dyes. Arrange the tumblers and bowls on the trays on top of a low table. Ensure that the children wash and dry their hands.

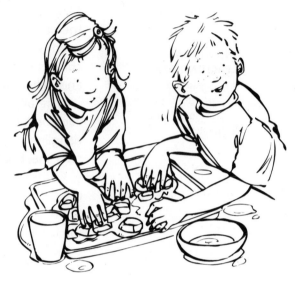

Bring in a tray of colourless ice. Loosen the ice under a tap and empty the cubes onto the trays. Ask questions such as, 'How do the ice cubes feel to touch as they slither and slide over the surface of the tray?', 'What is ice made from?', 'What will happen to the ice in the warm room?' and so on. Encourage the children to put the ice in the tumblers or bowls and place these in the sunshine or the shade, in a cool place or near the radiator. Whose ice is melting first? Add ice cubes to a glass of warm water and see what happens.

Now bring in the coloured ice cubes and encourage the children to add them to the tumblers of clear water and watch the water change colour as the ice cubes melt. What is happening?

Finally, enjoy making fruity ice cubes together by placing small pieces of fruit in the ice tray, filling up with fruit juice and then freezing. Enjoy sucking these on a hot day. (NB Check for any food allergies or dietary requirements.)

Special support
As you experiment, encourage the child that you are targeting to use the words 'wet', 'dry', 'cold' and 'hot'. Show them by practical example what these words mean. Look for opportunities later in the session to reinforce these words.

Extension
Let the children make their own fruity cocktails with coloured ice cubes, drinks and fruit.

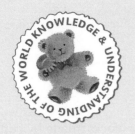

LEARNING OBJECTIVES FOR ALL THE CHILDREN
● to investigate materials by using all of their senses as appropriate
● to select the tools and techniques that they need to shape, assemble and join the materials that they are using.

INDIVIDUAL LEARNING TARGET
● to identify materials that are 'too big' or 'too small'.

Design a lorry

Group size
Three or four children.

What you need
Large sheets of sugar paper; glue; spreaders; large range of collage materials cut into squares, oblongs, circles and triangles in different sizes, colours and materials; tray; sticky tape; split-pin fasteners; stapler (adult use).

What to do
Arrange the collage materials on a tray. Sit down with the children and suggest that you make a truck with the materials. Talk together about the shapes and the materials as you work out which pieces to use for the body, the cab and the wheels of your vehicle. Show the children how to paste the collage together and be led by them if they suggest adding paint or felt-tipped-pen detailing. As you meet particular problems, such as how to stick on a plastic lid to make a wheel, or how to make a cardboard circle turn round, talk together about how you might best select and join the materials.

Special support
Offer the child that you are targeting a choice of pieces of materials and talk about which might be too big or too small. Let this conversation flow as naturally as possible between you as you select the best sized pieces for your collage.

Extension
Let the children use the collage materials to make three-dimensional lorries. Can they design them so that the wheels turn, too?

LINKS WITH HOME
Suggest that parents and carers carry out a clothes sorting activity with their children at home and that they ask questions such as, 'Which clothes are too big?', 'Which are too small?' and 'Which are just right?'.

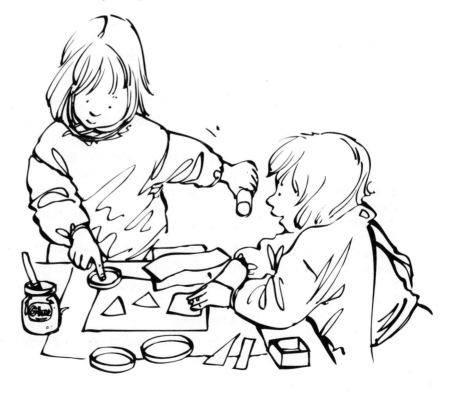

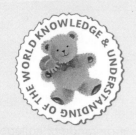

Gift wrap

Group size
Six to eight children at a time.

What you need
Large sheets of white paper; sponge printing blocks (made by cutting facets and patterns into sponge blocks); paint trays with diluted paint.

What to do
Arrange your materials on a table and gather the children around. Show them how they can dip their sponge printing blocks into the paint and make an impression on the paper. Demonstrate to the group how to make regular patterns while they watch, for example, a row of red prints at the bottom, then a row of blue and so on, or yellow circles and then yellow triangles.

Encourage each child to think of a pattern and then support them as they try to follow it through.

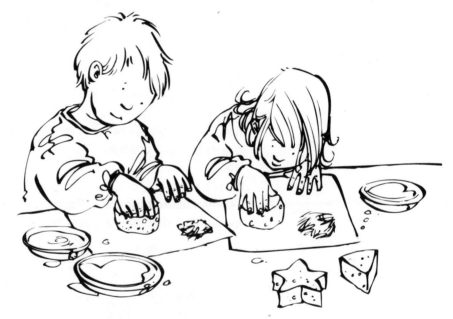

Special support
Use this activity to reinforce the child's understanding of colours. Concentrate on the four basic colours – red, green, blue and yellow. First, point to a colour print and ask the child that you are targeting to make another one the same. Note whether they can match each colour in this way. Now ask the child to make a red print. Observe whether the child can identify each colour in this way. Finally, ask the child to tell you the colour of a print that you point to. Keep a note of whether they can name each colour in this way. 'Teach to the gaps', starting with matching, then identifying, and finally naming. Use the activity to keep the conversation as natural as possible.

Extension
Let the children design sheets of paper to use as gift wrap for the particular occasion or festival.

LEARNING OBJECTIVE FOR ALL THE CHILDREN
● to look closely at similarities, differences, patterns and change.

INDIVIDUAL LEARNING TARGET
● to match, identify and name basic colours.

LINKS WITH HOME
Once you are 'teaching to the gaps', ask the parents or carers of the child that you are targeting to help their child bring in three things which are 'yellow' and so on.

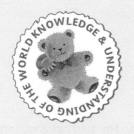

LEARNING OBJECTIVE FOR ALL THE CHILDREN

● to investigate foods using their sense of smell and taste.

INDIVIDUAL LEARNING TARGET

● to respond to the action words 'smell' and 'taste'.

Delectable delicacies

Group size
Whole group.

What you need
A selection of tastes and delicacies from several cultures represented in your community; relevant table decorations.

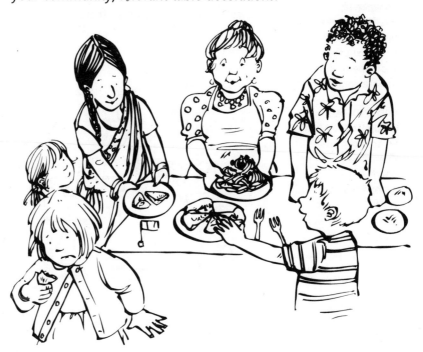

What to do
Plan this activity well in advance of carrying it out. Ask parents, carers and colleagues to help you to design a tasting session of different savouries, snacks and sweet things from their particular culture or favourite holiday destination. Start collecting table decorations, cloths, candles and fabrics that will accompany your feast. Talk to the children during the preparations so that the excitement and anticipation builds up. Send out invitations to parents and other special visitors who can contribute to your feast.

When the day comes, encourage the visitors to stand by their delicacies so that they can talk to the children about what they are. Each should be served in tiny portions for a child to smell or to taste. Encourage the children to experiment but warn everyone not to be offended if there are some wry faces! (NB Check for any food allergies or dietary requirements.) Send out 'thank you' letters to the visitors and helpers.

Special support
Ask the child's key worker to stay close to encourage the child to 'smell' and then to 'taste' if the smell was pleasing. Talk about which tastes and smells the child likes and which they do not. Do not force them to eat anything; you can still talk about the food.

Extension
Let the children help you to prepare some of the delicacies.

LINKS WITH HOME
Involve parents and carers from an early stage and ask them to help by sending in a range of tastes in line with your 'theme' or 'culture'.

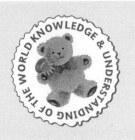

Grand prix

Group size
Whole group.

What you need
A remote-controlled or programmable vehicle toy such as a racing car or a truck with a simple operating pad; an outside playground or an indoor hall; chalk; egg timer or clockwork timer.

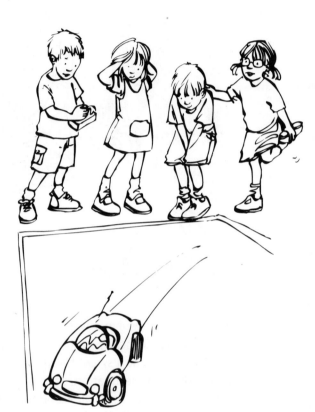

What to do
Encourage the child that you are targeting to choose a partner. Go with them to the space that you are using and show them how to operate the toy. Make any safety rules clear and define the space distinctly where the vehicle can go. Explain that if it goes outside that area, you will need to take the control pad back. Define the boundary of the area with chalk. Stay with the children all the time.

Provide hand-over-hand support to the child that you are targeting at first. Use the egg timer or clockwork timer to give each child a fair turn of three minutes. Once each child has had a turn, suggest a partner game in which one child calls 'Go' and 'Stop' while the other child operates the vehicle. Praise them for co-operating in this way. Continue until all the children have had turns, two at a time.

Special support
If you need to, whisper 'Go' and 'Stop' to the child that you are targeting to encourage them to give their partner directions at the correct time. Praise them for playing well with their partner.

Extension
Talk about radio-controlled and programmable toys and explain to the children in simple terms how they work. Arrange for some visitors to come to your setting to give a demonstration.

LEARNING OBJECTIVE FOR ALL THE CHILDREN
● to explore and experiment with a remote-controlled toy.

INDIVIDUAL LEARNING TARGETS
● to work co-operatively with a partner
● to speak out with confidence
● to use the words 'stop' and 'go'.

LINKS WITH HOME
Suggest that parents and carers play a 'Stop and go' game with their children on their way home, stopping safely at the kerbs.

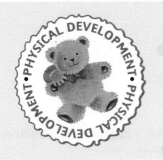

PHYSICAL DEVELOPMENT

This chapter encourages all the children's physical development. There are suggestions for supporting children who might find verbal instructions difficult and who might need practice in linking actions to words.

LEARNING OBJECTIVE FOR ALL THE CHILDREN
● to move hands with control and co-ordination.

INDIVIDUAL LEARNING TARGET
● to repeat a familiar phrase with confidence.

The big ship sails

Group size
Whole group.

What you need
A soft rope, approximately 1cm in diameter, long enough to go around the circle of children and knotted together to form a ring.

What to do
Ask the children to sit in a circle on the floor. Unfold the rope and pass it around so that each child is holding it with two hands. Demonstrate to the children how to pass the rope around the circle by shifting their hands and show them which way to pass it. Encourage them to practise doing this. Sing 'The Big Ship Sails Through the Alley, Alley O' (Traditional). You will find the tune in *This Little Puffin…* compiled by Elizabeth Matterson (Puffin Books).

The big ship sails through the Alley, Alley O;
Alley, Alley O; Alley, Alley O.
The big ship sails through the Alley, Alley O,
On the last day of September.
The captain said, 'It will never, never do;
(and so on)
The big ship sank to the bottom of the sea;
(and so on)
We all dip our heads in the deep blue sea;
(and so on)

At the end of each verse, pause to ask, 'Who has got the knot?' and to cheer that person.

Special support
Encourage the child that you are targeting to join in the refrain as well as they can. Sing other simple rhymes as they all tend to have refrains, for example, 'Old MacDonald Had a Farm'. Praise the child for calling their name out clearly when you ask and when they have the knot.

Extension
Use a thinner rope and thread a curtain ring onto it. Encourage older children to pass the ring under their hands and around the rope so that you cannot see who has the ring.

LINKS WITH HOME
Let the child that you are targeting take home rhymes with refrains to enjoy and practise with their family. Encourage the parents or carers to accept and praise any joining in at first, even if the words are not clear.

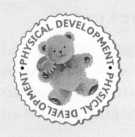

LEARNING OBJECTIVE FOR ALL THE CHILDREN
● to move with confidence and co-ordination.

INDIVIDUAL LEARNING TARGET
● to respond appropriately to the words 'high' and 'low'.

Dancing hands

Group size
Ten to 20 children.

What you need
A CD or tape of modern disco backing music (alternatively, switch on the rhythm section of an electronic keyboard).

What to do
Sit in a circle together on chairs. Tell the children that they are going to teach their hands to do a dance. Ask them for some ideas for hand movements and see whether they can build these into a 'rap'.

> Raise your hands up HIGH,
> Put your hands down LOW.
> Clap them FAST FAST FAST,
> Clap them SLOW SLOW SLOW.
> Raise your hands up HIGH,
> Put your hands down LOW.
> Clap them ONE, TWO, THREE,
> Make them GO GO GO!
>
> *Hannah Mortimer*

Practise the rap together and then try it with the backing music. Emphasize the key words loudly. Keep it fun and light-hearted and suggest that the children tell their hands how clever they have been!

Special support
Read the rhyme slowly. Prompt the child that you are targeting to join in with the hands high and hands low at the appropriate time by showing them what to do, by gently nudging their elbow or by providing hand-over-hand support. Always choose the prompt that provides the least help, to encourage the child to respond.

Extension
Invite the children to make up their own versions of the rap and teach them to the others.

LINKS WITH HOME
Let the child that you are targeting take home a final version of the rhyme to practise the words and actions with their parents or carers.

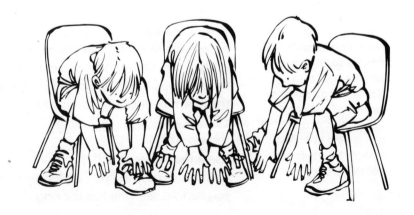

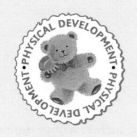

LEARNING OBJECTIVE FOR ALL THE CHILDREN

● to travel around and through equipment.

INDIVIDUAL LEARNING TARGET

● to respond appropriately to the words 'around' and 'through'.

LINKS WITH HOME

Ask the parents or carers of the child that you are targeting to practise the words 'through' and 'around' by playing a game at home with a teddy and a cardboard box.

Tunnel turns

Group size

Two or three children.

What you need

Three or four very large cardboard boxes from a supermarket; large scissors (adult use); a plastic play tunnel, if available; a large space on a smooth or carpeted floor suitable for crawling on.

What to do

Cut two openings at the ends of each cardboard box to make a tunnel large enough for a child to crawl through on opposite sides and at floor level. Make circular roof holes that let the light in and that are also large enough for the children to pop their heads out of. Arrange the boxes in a line with a child's height gap between them.

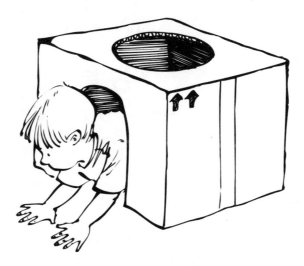

Invite the children to take turns to crawl through the tunnel and show them how to keep a safe distance between themselves. Encourage them to pop their heads out of the roof windows to let you know how far they have gone.

Now set each child a challenge while the others watch, by asking them to crawl *through* the first box, crawl *around* the second box, put their heads *through* the next window, and so on. Clap and celebrate each success.

Special support

Repeat the key words for the child that you are targeting so that they learn to link the words 'through' and 'around' with concrete actions. Focus their attention on the child performing the challenge and ask if that child is going *around* or *through* the boxes. Walk beside them as they try the challenge so that you can make sure that they understand the key words and ensure success.

Extension

Ask the children to help you draw where the openings should go on the boxes ready for you to cut out.

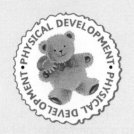

LEARNING OBJECTIVE FOR ALL THE CHILDREN
● to show awareness of space, of themselves and others.

INDIVIDUAL LEARNING TARGET
● to identify 'big' and 'small'.

Magic carpet

Group size
Six to 12 children.

What you need
A large mat which you can all sit on together, such as a floor rug or a PE safety mat; individual mats made from pieces of carpet squares or sheets of thick paper that the children have decorated themselves, one for each child; an open space.

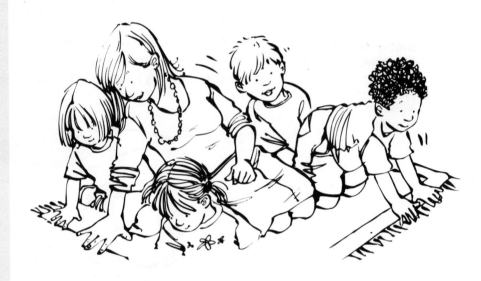

What to do
Gather the children on the big mat for a game of 'Pretend'. Say 'Wouldn't it be wonderful if the carpet could fly! Shall we pretend?'. Sit tight as you invent some magic words to say. Chant them together and provide a running commentary as you all hang on tight, for example, 'We are flying *this* way (all lean to the left) and *that* way (all lean to the right). Oh no! Now it's bumpy! What can you see down below?'. Develop the game by encouraging the children to think of their own ideas. Make sure that you land safely.

Now suggest to the children that they have their own magic carpets, and encourage each child to place their small mat in a space and sit on it as your story continues.

Finish with a final trip together on the big mat, repeating all your adventures in reverse order as you fly all the way home.

Special support
Throughout the game, provide directions to the child that you are targeting to go to the 'big' mat or to find their 'small' mat. Look for natural opportunities to reinforce these key words.

Extension
Encourage the children to retell their magic-carpet story for you to write down with them, and then ask them to illustrate it.

LINKS WITH HOME
Suggest to the parents or carers of the child that you are targeting to use the family's collection of shoes to practise talking about 'big' and 'small'.

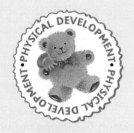

LEARNING OBJECTIVE FOR ALL THE CHILDREN
● to move with confidence and in safety.

INDIVIDUAL LEARNING TARGET
● to speak loudly when appropriate and with confidence.

Touch tig

Group size
An even number of children up to 12.

What you need
Brightly coloured chiffon scarves, one for each pair of children; a large open space; non-slip trainers or plimsolls.

What to do
Choose the child that you are targeting to show the other children what to do. Tuck a chiffon scarf lightly in your belt or waistband so that it hangs behind you. Ask the child to chase you and try to pull the scarf away. Tell them to shout 'Tig!' as they catch hold of it. Encourage everybody to cheer the child on, and make sure that you are indeed 'tigged'. Now tuck the scarf lightly into the child's waistband and chase them until you can catch it and shout 'Tig!'.

Pair the children up and ask them to come back to you each time one of them has 'tigged' the scarf so that you can say 'Well done' and reattach the scarf to their partner.

Special support
Keep watch over the child that you are targeting so that you can remind them to shout 'Tig!'. If there is a particular speech sound that you are targeting at that time, choose a new catchword that will help the child to practise that sound, for example, 'Zig!' or 'Fish!'.

Extension
Encourage the children to use the chiffon scarves to make up a colourful dance to music.

LINKS WITH HOME
Ask the parents or carers of the child that you are targeting to help them practise their 'loud' voice at home, for example, by shouting for someone in the family to come and have their tea.

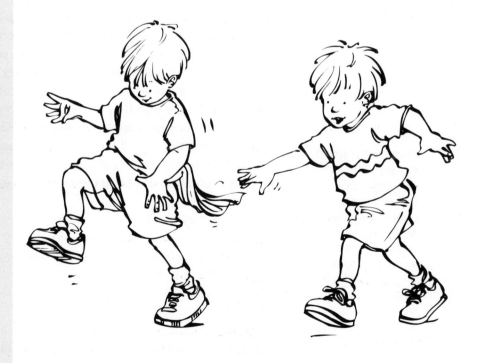

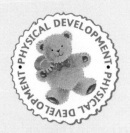

LEARNING OBJECTIVE FOR ALL THE CHILDREN
● to move with control and co-ordination.

INDIVIDUAL LEARNING TARGET
● to identify and to name colours.

LINKS WITH HOME
Ask the parents or carers of the child that you are targeting to send their child to the setting wearing several different colours. Encourage them to spend a little time talking to their child about the different colours that they are wearing.

Babbling brook

Group size
12 to 20 children.

What you need
An open space, approximately 20 metres between two opposite walls, such as in a playground or a school hall; brightly coloured PE bands or the children's T-shirts brought from home if the children wear uniforms.

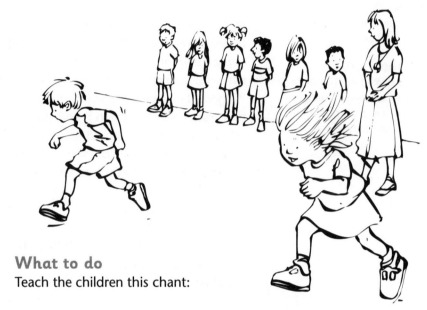

What to do
Teach the children this chant:

Babbling brook! Babbling brook!
May we swim across your water?

Invite the children to put on their T-shirts or brightly coloured bands and to stand along one of the wall. Take up a position in the centre, half-way between the two walls. Help the children to chant the refrain to you. Then answer, for example, 'Only if you are wearing *red* today!'. Encourage the children to look at what they are wearing and to run across to the other wall if they can find some red in their clothing. Invite them, whichever wall they are against, to repeat the refrain. Choose a new colour for your answer, for example, 'Only if you are wearing *blue* today'. The children will then be running across from both sides. Show them how to move safely at speed and praise them for not bumping into one another. Continue until you have exhausted all colours.

Special support
Invite the key worker to work alongside any children who are still learning their colours to help them look for and identify the colour you have called in their clothing.

Extension
Use different variations for the game, such as 'Only if your name begins with a "s"', 'Only if your birthday is in January', 'Only if you have brown hair' and so on.

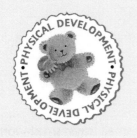

LEARNING OBJECTIVE FOR ALL THE CHILDREN
● to recognize the changes that happen to their bodies when they are active.

INDIVIDUAL LEARNING TARGET
● to develop an understanding of the word 'tired'.

LINKS WITH HOME
Give each child a copy of the photocopiable sheet on page 92 and encourage parents and carers to talk about it with their children at home.

Athletic antics

Group size
Ten to 12 children.

What you need
A large open space; non-slip trainers or plimsolls.

What to do
Gather the children together ready to go into the open space. Explain to them that they are going to think about what happens to their bodies when they run around. Firstly, ask the children to keep their bodies really calm. Invite them to walk very slowly and gently into the space and find somewhere to lie down. Quieten your voice to a whisper as you creep softly into the space.

When all the children are lying down, explain that you are going to ask some of them to stand up and run very quickly on the spot. Demonstrate to them what you mean. Then move around, touching half of the group on the shoulder, encouraging them to stand up and run very quickly on the spot. Clap your hands after 30 seconds and ask all the children to sit up.

Now talk about the differences between the two groups of children. What do they notice? Discuss how the children who were running are breathing faster. Perhaps they are red-faced because their hearts are working faster to push the blood around the body to give them more energy. Perhaps they are feeling tired. Now swap over groups, so that the children who ran on the spot now rest and the children that were lying down now run on the spot. After 30 seconds, compare the differences again.

Finish with an energetic game and then return to your usual area for a quiet activity.

Special support
Talk with the child that you are targeting about being tired. Ask them, 'What do you do at home when you are tired?'.

Extension
Share a simple picture book with the children about how our bodies work and how we make that sure we that have the energy to move.

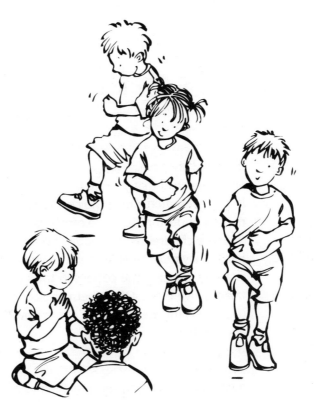

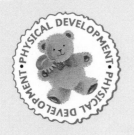

LEARNING OBJECTIVE FOR ALL THE CHILDREN
● to handle small objects with increasing control.

INDIVIDUAL LEARNING TARGET
● to respond appropriately to 'big', 'small' and to simple descriptions of colour and quantity.

LINKS WITH HOME
Try to link your theme to any important events in the children's lives, such as a visit to a hospital, a new play area, a space story on the news and so on.

It's a small world

Group size
Two children at first, then three or four.

What you need
A sand tray with sand; two small tables; two small trays; small-world play people and props such as a farmyard set, a Noah's ark set or sets from construction and imaginative play toys, for example, a zoo, space station, playground, hospital, school and so on.

What to do
Before the children arrive at your setting, place some of the items in the sand tray to fit in with the theme that you have set. Arrange them to give the children an idea of how they could lay them out. Place the other items in trays so that they can be clearly seen on two tables, one on each side of the sand tray. Ask the child that you are targeting to choose a partner who is happy to join them. Stay beside them as you tell the story

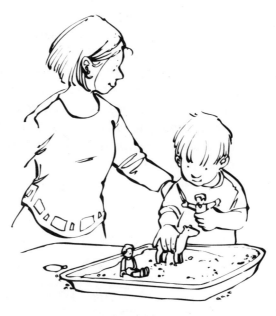

of the scene in the sand tray and support the children as they develop the game with the other items. Encourage them to ask appropriately for items that are within reach of the other child and to say 'Thank you'.

Step back as the game progresses, returning with new ideas if you need to. Gradually extend the time that you encourage the children to carry on playing. Let everyone have a turn if they want to. Choose a new theme the next session.

Special support
Show the child that you are targeting how to ask appropriately if they tend to grab or snatch. Praise the children for being helpful to one another. Find natural opportunities to reinforce concept words such as 'big' or 'red'.

Some children with language difficulty find imaginative play very hard. They may be able to play 'symbolically' with the toys, for example, placing the patient in the bed, but tend not to have new imaginative ideas. Offer them choices to extend their play, for example, 'Do you want the doctor to come now?', 'Is her Mum going to come and see her?' and so on.

Extension
Invite the children to suggest themes and to set up the activity.

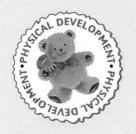

LEARNING OBJECTIVE FOR ALL THE CHILDREN
● to recognize the importance of keeping healthy and those things which contribute to this.

INDIVIDUAL LEARNING TARGET
● to join in with key action words.

Atishoo!

Group size
12 to 20 children.

What you need
A box of tissues; bin; plate of fresh fruit pieces; child-sized warm hat, gloves, coat and scarf.

What to do
Gather the children in a circle to sing 'Ring-o-Ring-o-Roses' (Traditional) and join hands. Move around the circle as you sing, crouching down on the last word and emphasizing the sneeze. Repeat the rhyme two or three times.

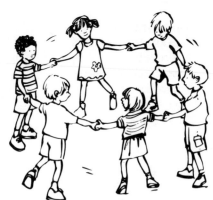

Pause to talk about colds and sneezes. Ask the group, 'What do you do when you need to blow your nose?'. Point out how 'a tissue' sounds the same as 'atishoo!'. Tell the children the second verse, sitting down in your circle.

> Polly's caught a cold now; She thinks she's going to sneeze now; A tissue! A tissue! To blow her nose!
>
> *Hannah Mortimer*

Pass a box of tissues around the circle so that everyone can pretend (or otherwise!) to blow their noses, and then go around with the bin to collect the tissues. Praise all the children for putting them in the bin. Talk about how to try not to catch colds. Pass around the plate of fruit pieces and talk about healthy foods. (NB Check for any food allergies or dietary requirements.) Pretend that it is a cold and windy day and invite a child to put on the winter clothes and talk about wrapping up warm.

Special support
Encourage the child that you are targeting to move downwards when you say the key word 'down'. Emphasize this word strongly. Some children with language difficulties find it hard to understand that words that sound the same can have different meanings, for example, 'a tissue' and 'atishoo!'. Talk about the two words and think of some others, for example, 'pail' and 'pale'.

Extension
Encourage the children to look after their own needs by using tissues and disposing of them appropriately. Have a special bin at 'cold' times and praise all the children for putting used tissue in there.

LINKS WITH HOME
Suggest to parents and carers that they help their children to choose extra warm clothing to come to your setting on winter days.

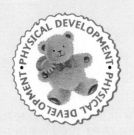

LEARNING OBJECTIVE FOR ALL THE CHILDREN

● to move the face with control and co-ordination.

INDIVIDUAL LEARNING TARGETS

● to blow
● to control tongue movements.

LINKS WITH HOME

Use the home/pre-school/therapist diary to keep in touch with the current therapy goals. If the therapist realizes how good you are at planning activities around the goals, then the flow of information will be much stronger. Use the diary to share the activity that you have carried out with the child that you are targeting with the parents or carers and the speech therapist.

Mirror, mirror

Group size
Two children.

What you need
A wall mirror; selection of funny hats.

What to do
Invite two children to join you for a game, including the child that you are targeting. Stand or sit in a line facing the mirror and choose a funny hat to wear. Now invite the children to look at you as you make a face, for example, purse your lips together, stick out your tongue, put your tongue to each side of your mouth and so on. Encourage the children to copy you and share the fun. Now ask the children to pair up and invite each child to copy the other, suggesting ideas if needed. Join in too, drawing attention to different face shapes and movements if it helps the other child to copy. Finish by each blowing on the mirror and drawing faces with your fingers in the steamed glass.

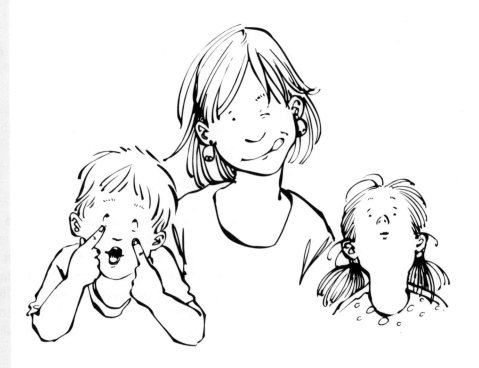

Special support
This activity might arise from knowing that there are certain mouth and tongue movements which the speech and language therapist wishes to encourage and practise with the child that you are targeting. They may need to learn to make blowing movements or to practise placing the tongue on the roof of the mouth, out in front, to the right or to the left.

Extension
Encourage pairs of children to mirror each other's movements by sitting opposite each other and copying. Practise blowing movements by using a straw to blow a coloured feather across a table in a 'feather race'.

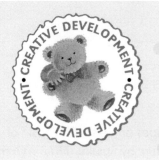

CREATIVE DEVELOPMENT

This chapter will help all the children to develop creatively. Ideas are also given for supporting children with speech and language difficulties through emphasizing key words and helping them to use words to plan and think.

LEARNING OBJECTIVES FOR ALL THE CHILDREN
● to recognize and explore how sounds can be changed
● to use their imagination in music.

INDIVIDUAL LEARNING TARGET
● to practise blowing.

LINKS WITH HOME
Let the child that you are targeting take home a selection of blowing toys and instruments to practise blowing. Encourage the parents or carers to play a game using a straw to blow a feather along. Give each child a copy of the photocopiable sheet on page 93 to take home and encourage them to describe the train journey in sounds to their parents or carers.

Runaway train

Group size
12 to 20 children.

What you need
Various percussion instruments, one for each child; large drum; whistle; CD player; 'Runaway Train' from *All Aboard the Runaway Train* (Jasmine).

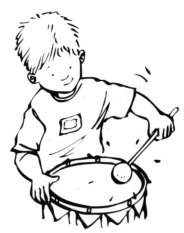

What to do
Invite each child to choose a percussion instrument. Make sure that the children understand how to play 'fast' and 'slow' by asking them to play 'fast' and 'slow' while you accompany them on a big drum.

Tell the children that you are going to play some train music. Pretend that the steam train has stopped in the station: 'Is everybody on board? Are all the doors closed? Here comes the guard, and she's going to blow her whistle! Count with me – one, two, three'. Give the child that you are targeting a whistle to blow.

Start very slowly and provide a running commentary: 'We're pulling out of the station – getting faster – very fast – here comes a hill – I think I can – over the hill and fast again – here comes a station – slowing down – all stop!' and so on. Repeat the blowing of the whistle when you start off again, and carry out the activity for two or three stations.

If you prefer, you can carry out this activity without music. Invite a few adults or older children to provide a strong beat, taking their lead from your percussion instrument. Include a strong drum, scratchy sounds and shaking sounds to give the impression of a train in motion.

Special support
Ask an adult to exaggerate 'slow' and 'fast' movements for the child that is being targeted while you teach the children how to play. Take a little time to practise blowing beforehand so that the child can show off this new skill. Blowing movements are important for the production of many speech sounds, but some children find mouth and air movements very difficult. Praise and encourage all their efforts.

Extension
Sit in a long line and pretend that you are the carriages. Encourage different children to be the guard, the driver and the passengers.

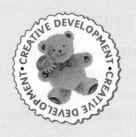

LEARNING OBJECTIVE FOR ALL THE CHILDREN
● to use their imagination in music and dance.

INDIVIDUAL LEARNING TARGET
● to use the words 'happy' and 'sad' appropriately.

Mood music

Group size
12 to 24 children.

What you need
CD player or tape recorder; selection of tapes or CDs with music of contrasting moods such as *William Tell Overture* by Rossini, *1812 – Overture* by Tchaikovsky and *Tubular Bells* by Mike Oldfield (Dabringhaus und Grimm); add ethnic music and modern music to reflect different cultures and tastes.

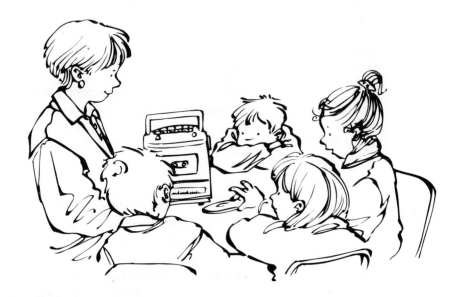

What to do
Before carrying out this activity, select about eight tracks or sections which you feel reflect very different moods and styles.

Invite the children to join you in an open space and play a short section of music. Stop it after 15 seconds or so and ask if the music makes the children feel 'happy' or 'sad'. Introduce new words as appropriate to the piece of music you have chosen such as 'angry', 'busy', 'peaceful' and so on. Always offer the children a choice of words. Invite the children to perform a 'sad', 'peaceful' or 'angry' dance as you replay the music for 30 seconds or so.

Repeat for each piece of music that you have chosen. In time, the children will suggest their own descriptions and can develop their own mood dances to suit the music.

Special support
Children with language difficulties may find this activity hard. Draw a set of pictures to represent happy, sad, angry, peaceful and busy people and use these to reinforce the choices of words that you are suggesting to them.

Extension
Invite the children to help you select the music and to tell you why they have made this choice.

LINKS WITH HOME
Ask the parents or carers of the child that you are targeting to talk with them and then to write down three things which make them feel sad and three things which make them feel very happy.

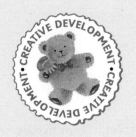

LEARNING OBJECTIVE FOR ALL THE CHILDREN
● to explore shape and texture in two dimensions.

INDIVIDUAL LEARNING TARGET
● to use simple descriptive words such as 'rough' or 'smooth'.

Touch talk

Group size
Four children.

What you need
The photocopiable sheet on page 94; an A3 piece of medium-textured sandpaper for each child (not too rough or too smooth); scissors; glue; cardboard box; tray to fit inside cardboard box; sticky tape.

What to do
Give each child an A3 copy of the photocopiable sheet and help them to glue it onto the smooth surface of the piece of sandpaper. Then help them to cut carefully around the outlines of each picture, taking care not to scratch themselves with the sandpaper. You will now have 16 sandpaper shapes, four of each kind.

Place the cardboard box on its side and use sticky tape to fix one of the side flaps down so that half of the opening is closed. Put this on a table and place four different shapes on the tray inside the box.

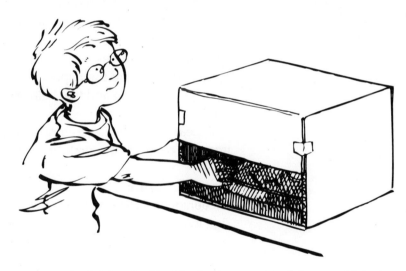

Invite each child to feel inside the box and to tell you which shape they have found before taking it out to see if they were correct.

Build up the number of pieces to choose from as the children become more proficient at touching and naming them. Play 'Find me one which is different' or 'Find me two which are the same' and so on.

Special support
Before you cut out the shapes, talk about the rough and smooth sides of the sandpaper. Practise naming each shape visually first so that you are sure that the child that you are targeting knows the name of each shape. When you use the box, have one of each shape on the table where the child can see them so that they remember what the choice is. Start with a choice of two shapes and gradually build up.

Extension
Encourage the children to use more complex and mathematical shapes such as stars, squares, circles, triangles and rectangles.

LINKS WITH HOME
Let the children take home the sandpaper shapes to show the guessing game to their parents or carers with their eyes shut or a scarf used as a blindfold.

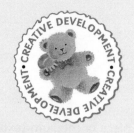

Five fat sausages

Group size
Ten to 15 children.

What you need
Old pairs of tights; soft tissue paper such as toilet rolls or tissues; scissors (adult use).

What to do
Before carrying out this activity, cut five leg lengths of tights and tie a knot in one end of each. Gather the children together in a circle and adapt the traditional chant 'Ten Fat Sausages' to:

> Five fat sausages sizzling in the pan,
> All of a sudden, one went BANG!
> Four fat sausages… (and so on)

Clap your hands loudly when you say 'bang!'.

Suggest to the children that you make some 'sausages' together to go with the rhyme. Show the group how to crumple the tissue paper and stuff it into the 'skin' to make a sausage. Encourage the children to work in twos or threes, with different children holding the 'sausage skin' open, crumpling up the paper and stuffing the paper into it. When the sausages are plump and full, help the children to tie another knot at the other end of each one.

Repeat the rhyme, each time inviting a child to take a 'sausage' away from the centre of the circle and another to count the remainder.

Special support
Encourage the children to say 'All gone!' at the end. Use the Makaton sign if the child that you are targeting is signing.

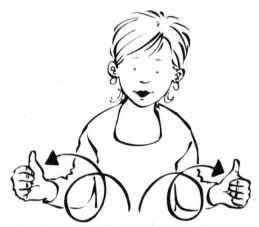

To finish

Extension
Invite the children to say the rhyme 'Ten Fat Sausages Sizzling in the Pan' in *This Little Puffin...* compiled by Elizabeth Matterson (Puffin Books). Count backwards in twos as the rhyme progresses.

LEARNING OBJECTIVES FOR ALL THE CHILDREN
● to explore texture and shape in three dimensions
● to respond in a variety of ways to what they touch and feel.

INDIVIDUAL LEARNING TARGETS
● to join in with a key word in a familiar rhyme
● to use the word 'gone'.

LINKS WITH HOME
'All gone' is a very useful and social early word for the child that you are targeting to learn. Ask the parents or carers to use the sign and word at all appropriate times, such as at the end of meals and when snacks have all gone.

78

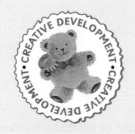

LEARNING OBJECTIVES FOR ALL THE CHILDREN
● to recognize and explore how sounds can be changed
● to use their imagination in music and story.

INDIVIDUAL LEARNING TARGETS
● to remember a sequence of sounds
● to link sounds to words.

Sea breezes

Group size
Groups of six children, each with an adult helper.

What you need
A selection of sound-making instruments (some can be purchased, such as rainmakers and ocean drums [see page 96] and maracas; others can be made, such as shakers, seed trays containing pulses [not red kidney beans] and tubes with rice or shale sealed inside); short video clip of the sea; large cockle shell, if available.

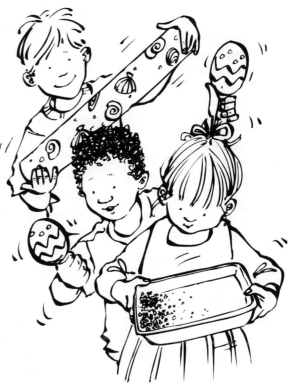

What to do
Gather the children together and talk about the sea. Establish which children have seen the sea and introduce the video clip if you feel that they are not familiar with the sounds of the sea. Pass around the cockle shell for the children to hold up to their ears, and praise them for listening so quietly. What can they hear?

Ask the children what kinds of sounds the sea might make. Talk about 'calm' sea and 'rough' sea. Play some of the instruments and ask the group to listen to them and say whether they sound a like the sea. Now invite the children to go into groups with their helper to choose instruments and make sounds with their voices that would be good sea noises. Suggest that the sea starts calm, then becomes rough and then calms again.

Let the children practise their sounds for five minutes in their individual groups, then ask them to come back together to listen to one another's sea sounds. Finish with a 'sound story' of the sea together.

Special support
Stay close to the child that you are targeting. Encourage them to remember the sequence of sounds from calm to rough to calm again. Praise them for looking at and listening to the other children.

Extension
Encourage the children to make a more elaborate and creative sound story of their own.

LINKS WITH HOME
Invite parents and carers to help their children make a sound-making instrument at home, such as a jar or bottle of rice, and bring it to your setting for a sound-effects story.

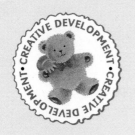

LEARNING OBJECTIVE FOR ALL THE CHILDREN
● to recognize repeated sounds and sound patterns.

INDIVIDUAL LEARNING TARGET
● to listen and repeat a percussion sound.

My turn, your turn

Group size
Ten to 20 children.

What you need
A large drum and two beaters (a large tambour or bodhrán is excellent, but other drums can be used instead).

What to do
Sit together in a circle on the floor. Carry out this activity at the beginning of circle time or music time as it works well as a greeting activity. Make a sound on the drum and then move around the inside of the circle as the children pass the beater to one another and take turns to bang it. Encourage them to make as loud a sound as possible the first time around the circle. Then invite them to make a very soft sound as you move around the circle a second time.

Now give each child a very simple rhythm to copy, for example, two beats, three beats, or a phrase, depending on each child's ability. Provide the rhythm with your beater and then hold the drum for each child to copy with the second beater.

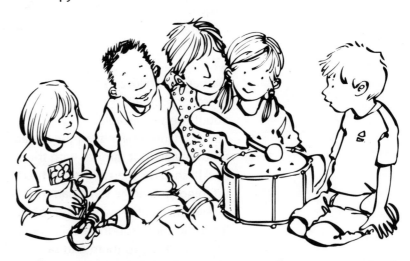

Finally, show the children how to beat their first names on the drum. Move around the circle saying 'Hello Phil-ip', 'Hello Car-ol-ine', 'Hello Ah-hyun' and so on, beating the syllables of the names as you say them. Then invite each child to copy with their beater as you repeat 'Hello...'.

Special support
Some children with language difficulties find reciprocal play – my turn, your turn – very difficult and this is a useful activity to practise the simple turn-taking involved in early conversations. They may need you to take the drum away after the correct number of beats and therefore succeed, with your help.

Extension
Some children will manage this activity independently and will not need to copy you when beating the syllables of their names. They might even be able to tackle, with practice, their full names or a phrase from a rhyme.

LINKS WITH HOME
Ask parents and carers to help their children clap the syllables of their first names at home.

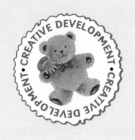

LEARNING OBJECTIVE FOR ALL THE CHILDREN
● to use imagination in their movement and role-play.

INDIVIDUAL LEARNING TARGETS
● to give eye contact
● to vocalize loudly.

Nursery howl

Group size
12 to 24 children.

What you need
Tape recorder; musical tape; range of percussion instruments; additional helper to operate the tape recorder.

What to do
Lead into this activity by starting with musical instruments. Encourage each child to choose an instrument and to march around in a circle as you start and stop the music. Each time you stop the music, give a new instruction such as 'Turn around and march the other way', 'Turn around in a circle' or 'Face the middle and march on the spot'. Each time you give a new instruction, show the children what to do. Then say 'Walk slowly into the middle and say "Hello!"'. Lead the children slowly in as the circle gets smaller and look at one another saying 'Hello!'. Stop the music, turn the children around and retreat back to the larger circle. Repeat this one more time.

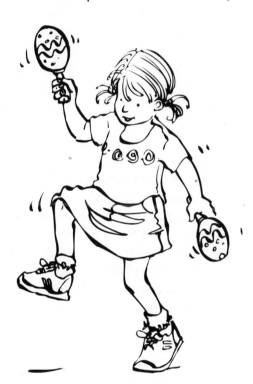

Now put your instruments away and join hands in a large circle. Ask the children to repeat what you do. Start with a low and a soft 'wooo' sound and move slowly into the middle of the circle. As you approach, raise your arms and the volume of your voice until you are all howling loudly in the centre of the circle with arms raised. Maintain eye contact with as many of the children as possible, with a smile and a nod of encouragement as you go. Retreat backwards slowly, lowering your voices again.

Special support
If the children are anxious, let them watch for the first few times and only join in when they feel ready. Place them next to you so that you can hold hands. This is a good activity for developing a 'group spirit' and practising voice modulation.

Extension
Make up a jungle howl chant with the older children and pretend to be wild animals roaring in a circle.

LINKS WITH HOME
Encourage the parents or carers of the child that you are targeting to make sure that they have eye contact from them when speaking or listening to them.

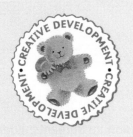

Under the sea

Group size
Three or four children.

What you need

A large rectangular box without a lid, for example, a Christmas-cracker box; blue Cellophane; cotton; scissors; different-coloured shiny or reflective card; shiny stickers; sequins; glue; spreaders; coloured tissue paper; paint; paintbrushes; felt-tipped pens; sticky tape; a picture book about the sea such as *Millie and the Mermaid* by Penny Ives (Puffin Books).

What to do

Read the picture book to the children and talk about the sea and the creatures that live there. Has anyone seen an aquarium? Suggest that you make your own aquarium full of brightly coloured fish.

Let the children mix different paint colours to find a greeny-blue 'sea' colour. Help them to paint the inside of the box but leave one of the long sides of the box unpainted – this will be the 'ceiling'. Place the box to one side to dry.

Then, help the children to glue the reflective sheets of card back to back so that there are two shiny sides, and place on one side to dry.

Invite the children to cut out long strands of 'seaweed' from the tissue paper. Then help each child to draw a fish shape with a felt-tipped pen on the reflective or shiny card and then cut it out. Show the children how they can select and stick on tiny sequins and stickers to decorate their fish. Leave these to dry.

When everyone has made a fish, attach cotton to them with sticky tape and suspend each one from the 'ceiling' of the box so that they turn and reflect light. Suspend strips of 'seaweed' from the ceiling. Finally, tape blue cellophane paper across the front to look like water.

Place your handmade 'aquarium' where the light will catch the fish. Admire the finished product together and encourage the group to talk about the effects.

Cellophane

Special support

Make sure that you practise language as you work together and talk about the colours and the textures of your creations. Emphasize action words clearly, for example, cutting, hanging, sticking, gluing and so on. The children will enjoy the finished effect of this activity.

Extension

Invite the children to help you design and assemble the aquarium.

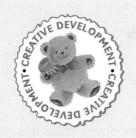

LEARNING OBJECTIVE FOR ALL THE CHILDREN
● to recognize and explore how sounds can be changed.

INDIVIDUAL LEARNING TARGETS
● to use non-verbal communication with confidence in a large group
● to look and to listen in a large group.

Band-time bonanza

Group size
12 to 24 children.

What you need
A selection of percussion instruments, for example, shakers, bells, drums, tambourines, wooden blocks and so on; CD player or tape recorder; musical tape or CD; a helper to operate the tape recorder or CD player.

What to do
Choose the instruments that you would like the children to play. Give them out in sections so that all the children with shakers are next to one another, then the drums, then the jingle bells and so on.

Tell the children that you are going to be the conductor and they must watch very carefully because you will show them when to start and when to stop. Introduce two hand signals – a downward arm movement for 'Start' and a policeman's halt signal for 'Stop'. Let the group practise starting and stopping to the appropriate signal.

Now tell the children that you will point to different groups of instruments and tell them when to start and stop. Ask your helper to start the tape or accompaniment, then signal to the drums, to the bells, to the shakers and so on when they are to join in and when they are to stop. Bring the groups of instruments in gradually and have a central section with everyone taking part, then gradually fade the music as different sections drop out again. Praise the children for watching you.

Special support
Arrange for an adult to sit next to the child that you are targeting so that the child's attention can be focused and their attempts encouraged.

Extension
Let the children perform this activity at an open day or concert, keeping it relaxed and happy. Introduce other hand signals to make it more challenging, for example, 'Start', 'Stop', 'Loud', 'Soft' and so on.

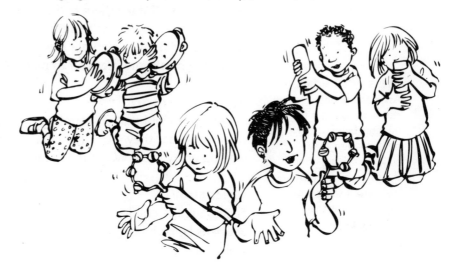

LINKS WITH HOME
Encourage the parents or carers of the child that you are targeting to come in to watch how well their child is looking and listening and to praise their progress.

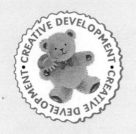

LEARNING OBJECTIVE FOR ALL THE CHILDREN
● to express and communicate their thoughts and feelings using a widening range of materials.

INDIVIDUAL LEARNING TARGET
● to talk about their session to a familiar adult.

LINKS WITH HOME
Ask parents and carers to spend a few minutes before bedtime with their children talking about their day, what went well and if there was anything that they felt sad about.

Good days, bad days

Group size
Two or three children.

What you need
Cardboard box with a clown's face on with his downturned mouth cut out to make a post-box (see below); paints; paintbrushes; paper; easels; felt-tipped pen.

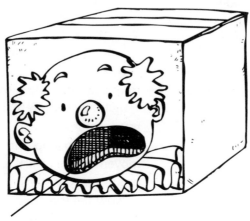

Cut out mouth to make post-box

What to do
Carry out this activity during the last half of the final session of the week, to review each child's progress throughout the week.

Invite the children to come to the easels to tell you about their week. What did they really enjoy doing at nursery? Encourage them to paint a picture of what they were really proud or happy about and talk with them about it. Write underneath the picture what they tell you.

Now ask the children if there was anything that they felt unhappy about or did not like. Was there anything that they want to do better? Prompt them gently to help them express themselves. Encourage them to paint a second picture, and write underneath what they tell you. Leave the paintings to dry.

Gather the children together just before home time and ask them if they would like to throw away their 'bad times' pictures. Unless they really do want to take them home, encourage each child to ceremoniously post their 'bad times' into the clown post-box and say 'goodbye' to them. Celebrate the 'good times' pictures and encourage the children to show these off to parents and carers as they arrive.

Special support
Support the child that you are targeting as they tell you about their week and what they did. Offer choices if necessary, for example, 'What did you enjoy best? Was it the painting or the slide?'.

Extension
Encourage the children to think more effectively about their early years activities by inviting them to plan and review their sessions regularly with you.

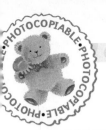

Individual education plan

Name:	Code of Practice Stage:
Nature of learning difficulty:	

Action	Who will do what?
1. Seeking further information	
2. Seeking training or support	
3. Observations and assessments	
4. Encouraging learning and development	

What exactly are the new skills we wish to teach?
How will we teach them?
What opportunities will we make for helping the child generalize and practise these skills throughout the session?
How will we make sure the child is fully included in the early years curriculum?
Help from parents or carers:
Targets for this term:
How will we measure whether we have achieved these?
Review meeting with parents or carers:
Who else to invite:

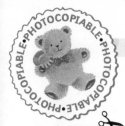

Smiles and frowns

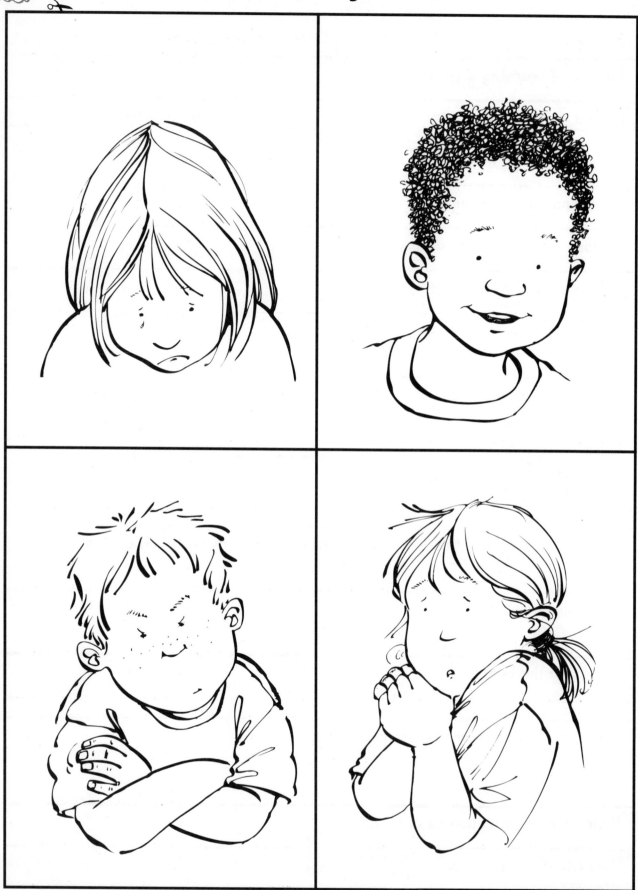

SPECIAL NEEDS **in the early years:** Speech and language difficulties

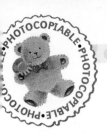

Now you see it

Play this guessing game with your child. Encourage them to help you cut out these pictures. Place the pictures on a table, then hide one. Can your child spot which picture is missing and describe it to you? If this is too difficult, hide pairs of matching pictures and build up the game.

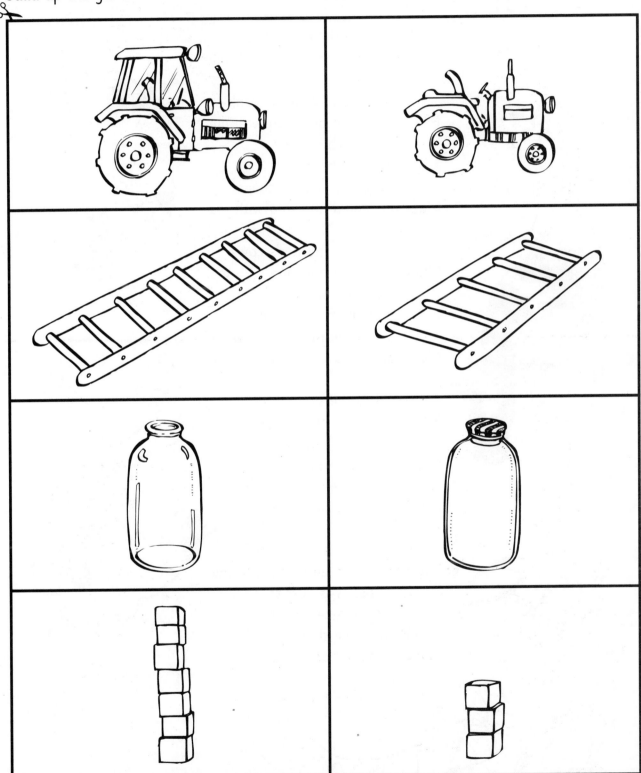

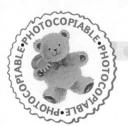

The buzzy bee song

(Tune: 'Twinkle, Twinkle, Little Star')

Listen to the buzzy bee!
Make the sound and sing with me:
zz-zz-zz-zz-zz-zz-zz
zz-zz-zz-zz-zz-zz-zz
Listen to the buzzy bee!
Make the sound and sing with me.

Listen to the woolly sheep!
Make the sound and sing with me:
b-b-b-b-b-b-baa
b-b-b-b-b-b-baa
Listen to the woolly sheep!
Make the sound and sing with me.

Listen to the farmer's cow!
Make the sound and sing with me:
m-m-m-m-m-m-moo
m-m-m-m-m-m-moo
Listen to the farmer's cow!
Make the sound and sing with me.

Listen to the singing birds!
Make the sound and sing with me:
la-la-la-la-la-la-la
la-la-la-la-la-la-la
Listen to the singing birds!
Make the sound and sing with me.

Listen to the slithery snake!
Make the sound and sing with me:
ss-ss-ss-ss-ss-ss-ss
ss-ss-ss-ss-ss-ss-ss
Listen to the slithery snake!
Make the sound and sing with me.

Hannah Mortimer

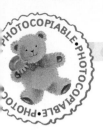

Story chains

Cut out these pictures and arrange them to make a story sequence.

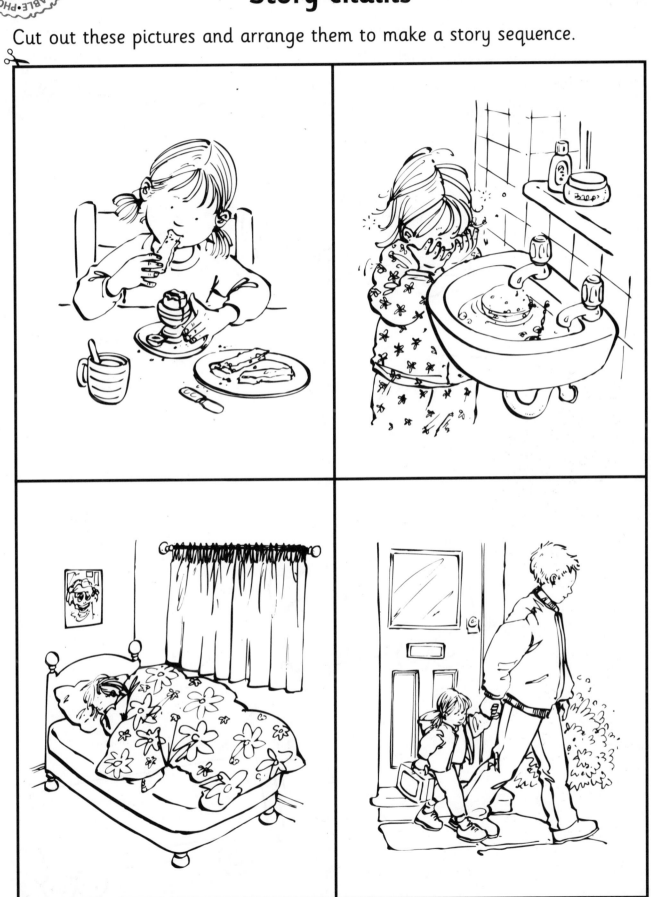

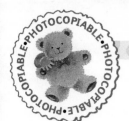

Tailback

Colour the *first* truck red.
Colour the *second* truck yellow.
What colour will you make the *middle* truck?
Colour the *fourth* truck green.
Colour the *last* truck blue.

SPECIAL NEEDS **in the early years:** Speech and language difficulties

Gone fishing

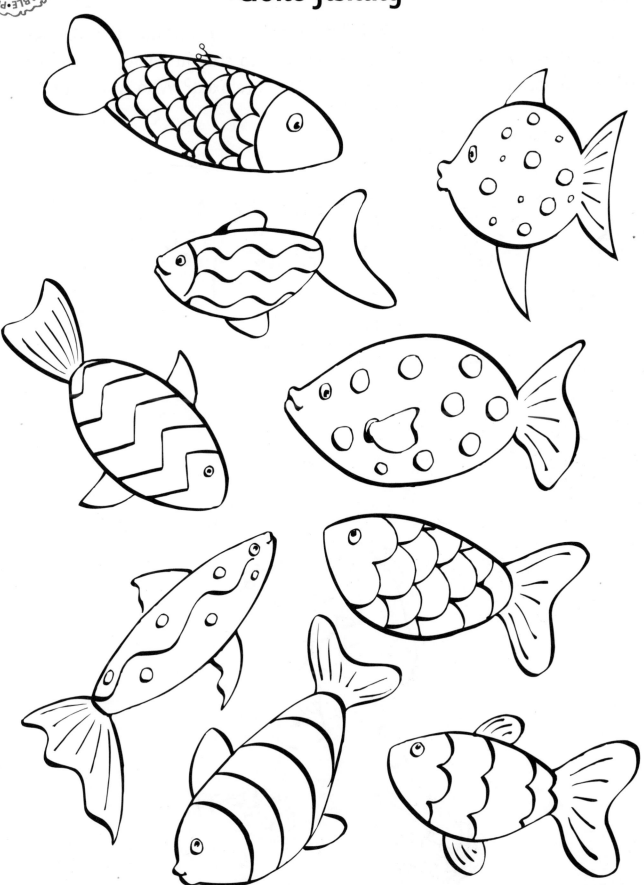

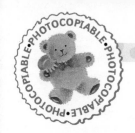

Athletic antics

Look at the children and spot the differences in the way that their bodies are working. We need to rest and to exercise to stay fit! Who is breathing faster? Whose heart is working hard? Who is relaxed? Who is happy?

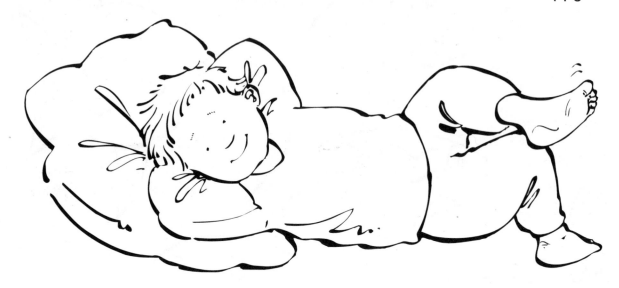

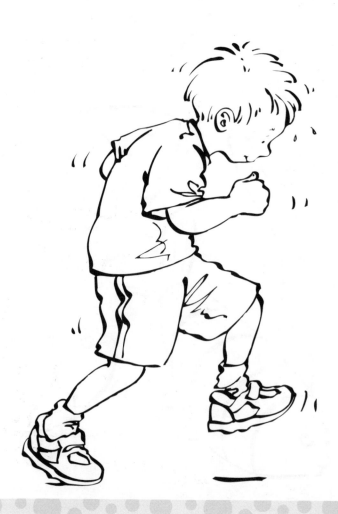

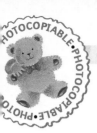

Runaway train

Make sounds to describe this train journey.

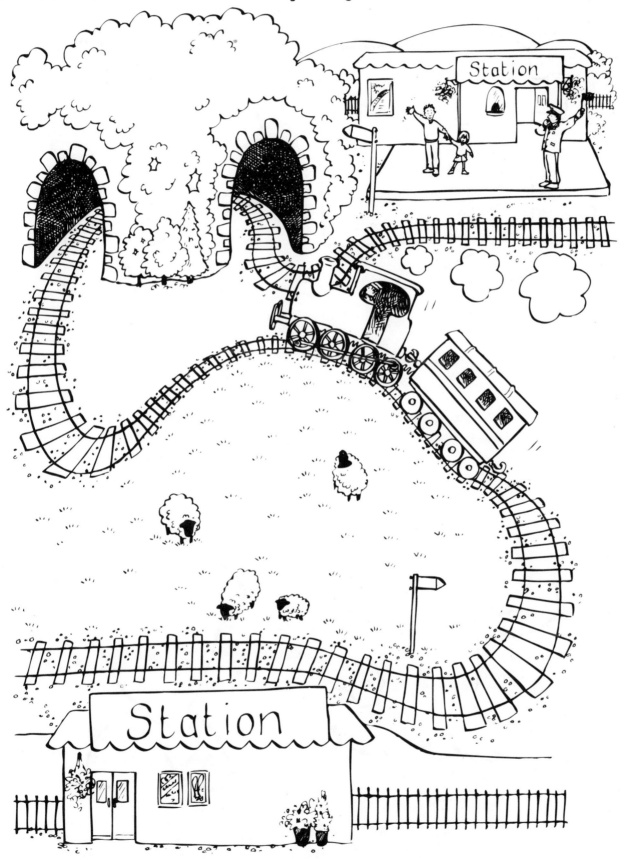

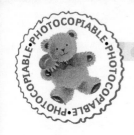

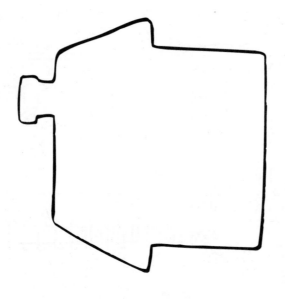

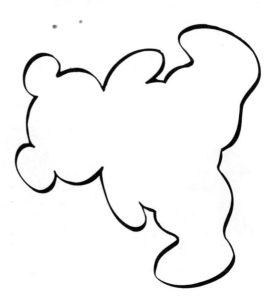

Touch talk

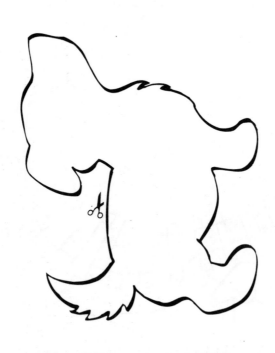

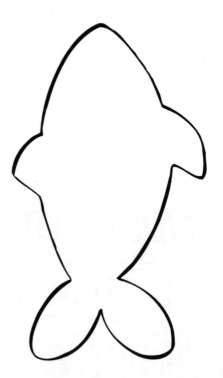

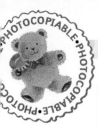

Under the sea

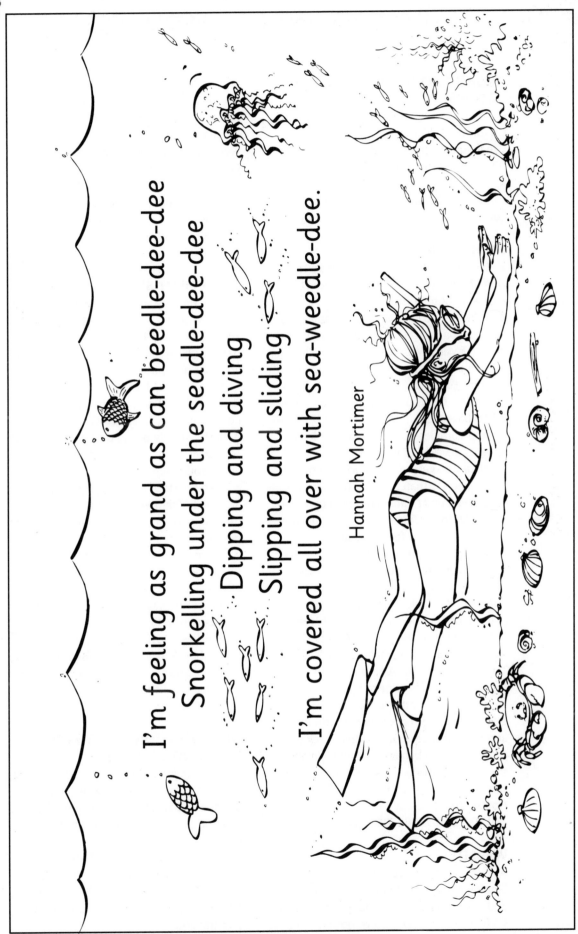

I'm feeling as grand as can beedle-dee-dee
Snorkelling under the seadle-dee-dee
Dipping and diving
Slipping and sliding
I'm covered all over with sea-weedle-dee.

Hannah Mortimer

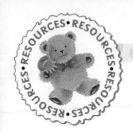

RECOMMENDED RESOURCES

ORGANIZATIONS AND SUPPORT GROUPS

● Association for All Speech Impaired Children (AFASIC), Second Floor, 50–52 Great Sutton Street, London EC1V 0DJ. Tel: 020-74909410.

● The Royal College of Speech and Language Therapists, 2 White Hart Yard, London SE1 1NX. Tel: 020-73781200.

BOOKS FOR ADULTS

● *Children's Language and Communication Difficulties* by Julie Dockrell and David Messer (Continuum)

● *Index for Inclusion: Developing Learning and Participation in Schools* by Booth, Ainscow, Black-Hawkins, Vaughan and Shaw (CSIE). Available from the Centre for Studies on Inclusive Education, Room 2S203, 5 Block, Frenchay Campus, Coldharbour Lane, Bristol BS16 1QU. Tel: 0117-3444007. Step-by-step considerations for a setting looking towards developing inclusion.

● *What Works in Inclusive Education?* by Judy Sebba and Darshan Sachdev (Barnardo's)

● *Oranges and Lemons* compiled by Karen King (Oxford University Press). Action rhymes and songs for music time.

● *The Music Makers Approach: Inclusive Activities for Young Children with Special Educational Needs* by Hannah Mortimer (NASEN). Available from NASEN (National Association for Special Educational Needs), 4–5 Amber Business Village, Amber Close, Amington, Tamworth, Staffordshire B77 4RP. Tel: 01827-311500. Advice on planning a regular music circle time to include children with speech and other difficulties.

● The *CaF Directory* of specific conditions and rare syndromes in children (including those that affect behaviour) with their family support networks can be obtained on subscription from Contact a Family, Equity House, 209-211 City Road, London EC1V 1JN. Tel: 020-76088700.

WEBSITES

● The Department for Education and Employment (DfEE) (for parent information and Government advice including the SEN *Code of Practice*): www.dfee.gov.uk

● The National Autistic Society (this is useful if the child has communication difficulties associated with a speech and language disorder): www.oneworld.org/autism_uk/nas (Tel: 020-79033555)

● The Writers' Press, USA, publish a number of books for young children about a range of SEN: www.writerspress.com

● The Hanen Centre (parent training and publications): www.hanen.org

EQUIPMENT SUPPLIERS

● LDA Primary and Special Needs, Duke Street, Wisbech, Cambridgeshire PE13 2AE. Tel: 01945-463441. Supply a range of pencil grips, language card, listening activities and puppets.

● NES Arnold, Novara House, Excelsior Road, Ashby Park, Ashby de la Zouch, Leicestershire LE65 1NG. Tel: 01530-418901. Supply ocean drums and a range of special needs and language equipment and resources.

● Step by Step, Lee Fold, Hyde, Cheshire SK14 4LL. Tel: 0845-3001089. Supply toys for role-play and multicultural language development.

● Acorn Educational Ltd, 32 Queen Eleanor Road, Geddington, Kettering, Northants. NN14 1AY. Tel: 01536-400212. Supply small-world play toys and resources for language development.

● Winslow, Goyt Side Road, Chesterfield, Derbyshire S40 2PH. Tel: 0845-9211777. Supply 'Snooky the Snail's Pre-school Fluency Worksheets' and 'The Mighty Mouth Game'.

ORGANIZATIONS THAT PROVIDE TRAINING COURSES

● I CAN Training Centre, 4 Dyer's Building, Holborn, London EC1N 2QP. Tel: 0870-0104066. Day courses available for those working with language-impaired children from early years upwards.

● Makaton Vocabulary Development Project, 31 Firwood Drive, Camberley, Surrey GU15 3QD. Tel: 01276-671368. Information about Makaton sign vocabulary and training.